OPERATION HOPE

Alzheimer's? Dementia? Cognitive Decline?
8 Pillars to Live Healthier, Stronger, Longer

OPERATION HOPE

Alzheimer's? Dementia? Cognitive Decline?
8 Pillars to Live Healthier, Stronger, Longer

ANN-LOUISE JOHNSON, IFMCP, RN

Copyright © 2018 Ann-Louise Johnson

Operation Hope: Alzheimer's? Dementia? Cognitive Decline? 8 Pillars to Live Healthier, Stronger, Longer

Ann L. Johnson
1135 Georgetown Road
Suite 120
Christiana, PA 17509
717-786-4798

Ordering Information:
Special discounts are available on quantity purchases by corporations, associations, and others. For details, contact the publisher at the address above.

www.dnaofhope.com | www.annljohnson.com

Orders by US trade bookstores and wholesalers.

Printed in the United States of America
First Printing, 2018

ISBN-13 (Paperback): 978-1-64255-160-0
ISBN-13 (Hardcover): 978-1-64255-161-7
ISBN-13 (Createspace): 978-1986649858
ISBN-10 (Createspace): 1986649857
ASIN: B0782RXXN9

NOTE TO READER:

This book was not written as a medical argument or to preach scientific jargon. Rather, it is a story about things that really matter—your life, your family, and your happiness. I spent forty years standing in front of patients in despair. And I found the medicine of hope to be as strong as any pharmaceutical development. With hope, many become victorious. I hope that after reading this book, you will join the ranks of victors.

DEDICATIONS

My clients. Thank you for holding on until I found you.

My parents. Dad, thank you for blessing me with your mantle of courage and adventure. Mom, thank you for the incredible gift of reading, and the hope reading grows.

My siblings. Perry and Priscilla, my brother and sister, and to the nine hearts that didn't make it to this life, but made it into my heart. Forever isn't long enough to love you.

My readers. With this book in hand, light the eternal flame within you. The flame of hope, yes, Operation Hope.

ACKNOWLEDGEMENTS

With marvel and joy, I acknowledge the following professionals: Rita M. Rhoads, CNP, MPH; Anna B. Morris, Health Coach; Deborah A. Everett, longtime friend and mentor; Arlene Weaver, hero and friend; Jeffrey Bland, PhD; Peter D'Adamo, ND; David Jones, MD; Ben Lynch, ND; Bernarda Zenker, MD; Mark Houston, MD; Dale Bredesen, MD; Robert K. Naviaux, MD, PhD; and Andreas Wagner, PhD.

TABLE OF CONTENTS

ABOUT THE AUTHOR

Scientist, adventurer, medical professional, and internationally known expert in healthy aging, Ann-Louise Johnson is the creator and founder of WildHeart Strong LLC, which teaches people how to age fiercely—to live life as an exciting adventure, and feel healthier, stronger, and more vital at every age.

For Ann, just being here is a miracle: she was one of only three children who lived after her parents' first nine children died immediately after birth. She grew up with two driving passions: the outdoors, where she always felt at home, and science. Ann wanted to know why she had survived while those other children had died.

She wanted to discover what causes people to get sick or to be healthy. As a registered nurse for 40 years, Ann worked both sides of the 911 call. "As a critical care nurse in trauma and intensive care units, I worked with accident victims and people with life-threatening [and often life-ending] illnesses," she says. "But eventually I wanted to see if I could keep people out of the ER by helping them stay healthier longer."

She accepted a position in one of the largest retirement communities in Pennsylvania, eventually becoming the director. It was there that an encounter with a 90-year-old warrior inspired Ann's groundbreaking research into successful aging. Ann discovered the difference between those who ended up incapacitated and in nursing homes and those who were still running marathons in their 80s was physical, mental, and emotional fitness.

She was first in her area to work with hundreds of people ages 60-90 to strengthen their muscles as well as their minds and attitudes, helping them reverse the effects of aging and live healthier, longer, stronger lives. Her results led her to speak at medical and professional conferences all over the world.

In 2011, Ann founded WildHeart Strong, a company that helps people change the way they age and rewrites the last half of their life story, changing it from a fear of aging to aging fiercely. Ann uses the latest scientific research in molecular biology and biochemistry, combined with practical functional medicine principles, and cutting-edge work in mental and emotional fitness, to create personalized health plans for clients of any age and fitness level. And because aging fiercely is not just about health, but about what you can do with stronger health, Ann leads WildHeart Strong adventures that crystallize these plans into daily life, providing exhilarating, instructive, and awe-inspiring experiences that many clients have only dreamed about.

Everything from snorkeling and scuba diving in the Caribbean to an International Space Station visit is on the WildHeart Strong "bucket list." "To be WildHeart Strong means to believe that life is an amazing adventure, a journey of exploration, discovery, and experience," Ann says. "It's an attitude and a mindset that pushes you and stretches you beyond the realm of normal experience into a new place of wonder and awe." Ann's step-by-step curriculum shows how you can change the way you age. Anyone can reverse the effects of aging, live life as an exciting adventure, and feel healthier, stronger, and more vital.

In 2013, Ann created and founded Younitype™ to educate clients about DNA, genes, and personalized biochemistry that can boost health. Younitype™, the name, captures the power of genes in what scientists call our genotype and the performance of those genes, called our phenotype. You have the power to boost your performance and empower some genes to work for you. Do you know your Younitype™?

It starts with a journey into your 8 Genomic Triggers. Know these eight; implement an action plan to boost these eight; personalize it by matching it to your specific genetic, biochemical, and lifestyle information. This is a lifelong tactical strategy for best health. And it's for the strong of heart, the courageous, the warriors, and those looking for hope again.

Ann is a Certified Functional Medicine Practitioner (IFMCP) and in 2017 received her Advanced Practice Certification in Reversing Cognitive Decline. What an exciting time to live! We can reverse many complex illnesses, including cognitive decline. Yes, we can create a new body within us. Our body can circumvent the current path of our sickness and build highways to health. This gives hope.

And this is why Ann created *Operation Hope: Alzheimer's? Dementia? Cognitive Decline? 8 Pillars to Healthier, Stronger, Longer*. We have been stumbling over the truth for years, but with recent molecular and genomic breakthroughs, we now have answers. Motivating answers like:

We can grow new neurons. We can grow healthier brain cells. We can create new neuron-synapse connections. We can remove toxic substances from the brain, including glucose. We can. Together we can. We have a second chance. Reversing cognitive decline takes a village, a support team. And in Operation Hope we build that team together. Reversing cognitive decline takes a whole new support team - the cells and genes within - our **Inside** Support Team. Oh! the wonders we find within each cell to ignite flames of recovery and health again. Let's start the journey...

CHAPTER ONE
WELCOME TO OPERATION HOPE

Imagine a woman. Imagine knowing this woman's life story—her strengths, triumphs, brilliance, gifts, and contributions to others, as well as to society overall. Imagine cherishing her with all your heart. Imagine that she is your mother.

And as you approach her with thousands of jumbled emotions all bunched up in your heart, see her beautiful eyes look back at you… blank and empty, as if someone, or something, had stolen the vibrant, brilliant person she once was and left only a shell to remain. She's there, but she's not. And while you are grateful that you can still be with her, still hug her, still tell her that you love her… you can't help but miss the person she once was, and to crave—just one more time—for her eyes to look back at you with the understanding, strength, and the sort of unspoken love that only your mother could share.

This is what it means and what it feels like to have a parent suffering from Alzheimer's, dementia, or cognitive decline. These silent diseases are not often talked about, or even thought about… until you are the child, longing for the parent you once knew.

However, cognitive disorders are on the rise.

By 2050, the number of people living with Alzheimer's is projected to grow to 160 million new cases, globally.

Stop and think about that for a second. *160 million people diagnosed with Alzheimer's by 2050.*

These are staggering numbers. And they are unacceptable numbers.

Our elderly are stripped of their memory, stripped of their abilities to do basic tasks. They lose their words. They are ostracized, and in return they ostracize themselves. Their world gets smaller and smaller. They stop going out into public for even simple tasks, for fear they will no longer recognize the faces of friends and associates.

Because we don't think of Alzheimer's as a curable disease, we unknowingly allow those who suffer from it to make it worse— through unhealthy diets, lack of brain stimulation, and an overall solitary existence.

Cognitive disorders are one of the greatest threats of today. They are the misunderstood, silent thieves of our quality of life. They are diseases that we have not previously understood and therefore have been accepted as an unfortunate potential part of life. What's worse? These diseases are quickly escalating from personal tragedy to societal tragedy. Soon it will not just be a problem for the unseen and unheard; it will something that touches almost all of us in one way or another.

It doesn't have to be this way.

Today, there is a new brand of researchers who refuse to allow such pain to continue unchallenged. There is a new thinking. A new possibility...

- What if we changed our mindset and our beliefs about cognitive disorders?

- What if Alzheimer's was a form of cancer, at the molecular level?

- And what if scientists were making headway in regenerating those abnormal molecules?

- What if it was possible to actually grow new brain cells? To grow new neurons? And to stimulate new synapses?

I have news for you—this is not science-fiction. This is where we are heading, and what is possible right now.

However, without a concerted, unified effort to prevent, or at a minimum to delay, the onset of Alzheimer's, this disease will become something we will no longer be able to ignore. There is a tidal wave approaching. If millions of people per year will soon be facing cognitive disease, who will get the care? And how will this impact our already unstable healthcare system?

The cruelty and pervasiveness of this disease demand a movement—that is, enough people with the courage to *believe* in what is possible. And to actually apply these new scientific breakthroughs with faith and steadfast determination.

It's easy to look the other way—to feel sorry for those whom this affects—and to pray that it never happens to us.

Until that person becomes your parent. And until you accept that we often live into our family trends and that you may be next to suffer.

My message today is about HOPE.

Hope for your parents.

Hope for your family and friends.

Hope for you.

New genomic studies now prove that these diseases CAN be reversed—and even better—prevented. Genomic scientific studies show our genes are influenced by our environment—meaning the food we eat, the air we breathe, the toxins we are exposed to, etc. **And right now, we are living in the era of a new genomic frontier—we are only at the forefront of understanding how incredible the inner genius that makes up each and every one of our cells is.**

Of the 25,000 genes we recognize, we know what just 2% of them can do. And it is powerful. These genes are responsible for creating the proteins and enzymes that act as building blocks for the rest of our body. They interact directly with the nutrients, emotions, and/or toxins that we put in our body every day to build and replenish, or break down our cells. Therefore, our genes, while containing a blueprint for whom we can become— are **not our destiny.**

This science is known as "nutrigenomics." This can start to feel complicated and confusing, but it's not. Here's the bottom line—our genes have triggers, known as "epigenomics," that can dim or brighten certain functions, and these triggers are influenced by what we consume and put into our bodies. And here's what that means—we're not treating or changing our genes themselves—rather, we have figured out how to change the *function* of our genes. We can now see how to turn down the dial on certain weakening functions, and how to turn up the dial on strengthening, health-inducing functions.

There is still hope in the fight against cognitive disorders… and this is a *big deal*.

Why? Because it puts "US" in the driver's seat. We do not have to be silent victims of the diseases we have previously tolerated and complied with. We have a choice. We have an opportunity to fight back, to rebuild the memories of our loved ones and build a defense mechanism to prevent our own memories from being lost in the first place. We can reverse and prevent modern illnesses—including the toughest and those previously thought impossible to cure.

The inside-workings of our DNA and cellular make-up are dynamic and tightly interwoven. Inside, we are like a huge spiderweb of DNA-cellular-mitochondrial and neuron-synapse connections. And we have the power to change the dynamics of illness at THIS cellular level to the dynamics of wellness.

Over the course of this program, I will walk you through a plan—a proven plan—to turn back the clock of cognitive decline for you, your loved ones, and anyone you may be caring for with a debilitating condition.

And remember as you take in each chapter,

Hope will carry your load…. when you've done all you can do.

And at the moment you want to give up on Hope, Hope will never give up on you.

Ann

CHAPTER ONE REFERENCES

Egan M, Bérubé D, Racine G, Leonard C, Rochon E. Methods to Enhance Verbal Communication between Individuals with Alzheimer's Disease and Their Formal and Informal Caregivers: A Systematic Review. International Journal of Alzheimer's Disease. 2010; 2010:906818. doi:10.4061/2010/906818.

Kempermann G, Song H, Gage FH. Neurogenesis in the Adult Hippocampus. Cold Spring Harbor Perspectives in Biology. 2015; 7(9):a018812. doi:10.1101/cshperspect.a018812. BMC Medicine. 2013 Apr 29; 11:115.

Rühli FJ, Henneberg M. New perspectives on evolutionary medicine: the relevance of microevolution for human health and disease. BMC Medicine. 2013; 11:115. doi:10.1186/1741-7015-11-115.

Hebert LE, Beckett L, Scherr PA, Evans DA. Annual Incidence of Alzheimer Disease in the United States Projected to the Years 2000 Through 2050. Alzheimer Disease & Associated Disorders. 2001 Oct-Dec; 15(4):169-173.

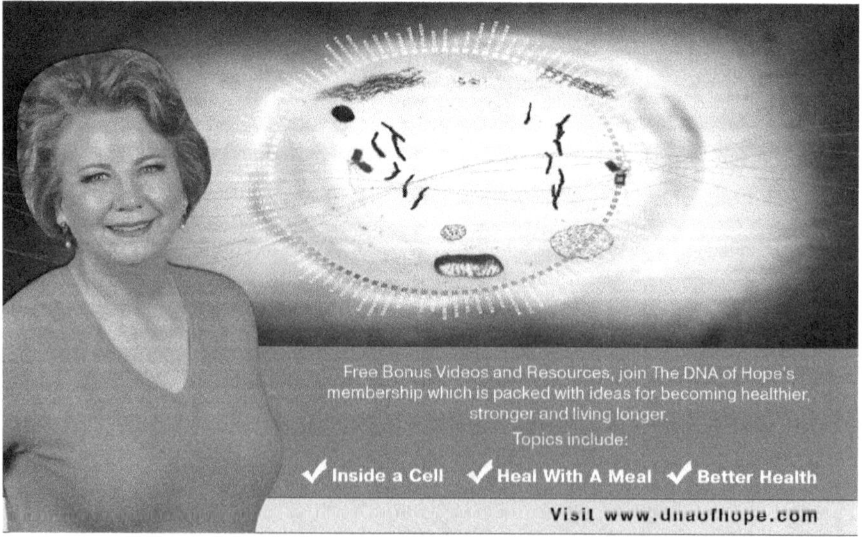

CHAPTER TWO
THE 8 PILLARS

There is a medicine of Hope inside of you: It is called the 8 Pillars. These Pillars are our lifestyle and habits and they help us stand up and fight this war against Alzheimer's and cognitive decline.

Let's briefly dive into each one of these, to help constructively paint a picture of how each one can impact your well-being—in both the short- and long-term. **In the process, I'd like to share just a few things you can do today—right now!—to program your DNA/genes for health.**

I really want you to see how each pillar affects you. Pay close attention, especially to your mental clarity and focus, after applying the techniques I am about to share.

PILLAR 1: SUPPORT

Although we crave support and care from each other, we don't necessarily realize that having it, or not having it, can impact how our DNA operates. Babies who are not nuzzled and held enough will literally stop growing. And if the situation continues, they will actually die—even if they are receiving all the nutrients needed to sustain life. This condition is known as "failure to thrive."

Even as adults, the attention and love that we receive from those around us still impacts us at a cellular level.

Being touched and nurtured is part of how we grow and evolve as a species. Without it, a part of our DNA is turned off—and our health declines as a result.

Neurons and synapses need external stimuli from friends and family to fire, as well. When someone begins to slip away into cognitive decline, our tendency is to stop reaching out, to stop communicating and spending time with that person... because it feels as if our efforts are futile. We don't think they can understand us anymore, and it's frustrating and scary to lose someone this way. So we leave them alone and isolated.

This is essentially like trying to heal an atrophied arm muscle... without moving it.

When a person's brain is not used, his or her synapses actually retract. It's like the inside of his or her body is screaming for support, but no one is listening. In order to stimulate the brain and help it repair itself, the brain's neural connections must be used and fired... And family and friends are a huge part of this type of rehabilitation. Even if a person doesn't make accurate connections immediately, the process of simply exercising those synapses through communication and support helps the brain rebuild.

PILLAR 2: MOTIVATION

What is motivation, really? It's this internal force that prompts a person to take action. It is what gives you power when you are at your weakest. It's a determination, a drive, a pursuit of a goal, no matter what—in the face of obstacles, boredom, fatigue, stress... and illness. **It is fuel for the eternal engine of hope.** But how does it impact our cells? Motivation releases endorphins, otherwise known as the "feel good" hormone in our brains. By continually associating to those aspects of life that inspire us to "act" and "do" by our own free will, we release chemicals that actually turn on positive DNA attributes. In fact, biologically-speaking, motivation impacts every neuron and synapse connection within you.

What motivates you? What inspires you to be your best? What will you fight for?

This insight—this passion—is literally a fuel that you can ignite throughout your mind, and throughout your body. By associating to this energy, you are essentially pouring growth hormone all over your neurons… stimulating new connections and enhanced brain power.

PILLAR 3: FOOD

Food is probably the most talked-about, MISunderstood—and definitely underutilized—genomic pillar. I could spend the rest of my time with you analyzing specific foods that either promote or negate health. However, for the purpose of this overview— here is what I think is most important for you to understand— foods that trigger a negative hormonal response will also trigger negative genomic consequences. Foods that trigger healthy and balanced hormonal cues will also trigger positive genomic consequences.

Now that may not mean a lot to you, as you may not understand how your hormones operate exactly. Hormones are basically signals that tell pretty much every function in your body what to do. And they are extremely potent. As an example, the amount of estrogen that would fit onto the tip of a pen is reactive enough to signal a woman's reproductive cycle. Our body keeps the rest in essentially a cage, to regulate how much is released and when. However, all of these signals can be influenced, and/or confused, by the types of foods we eat.

The most powerful hormone trigger, and the one that most of us know at least a little bit about—is glucose. Glucose is an energy regulator, and when it is raised too quickly, it confuses and overworks many other parts of our system. Therefore, the foods that too quickly elevate your glucose are also the foods that amplify degenerative functions in your genes. Specifically, those foods are sugars. All of the white stuff: bread, flour, rice, whole milk, packaged food, soda, sweets, and the most evil of all, high fructose corn syrup. These are "empty" carbs—the foods that spike your blood sugar (glucose), but that do not have any other nutrients or substances that your body can actually use to build and enhance your cells.

To date, processed, empty, sugary foods make up 70% of the U.S. diet.

70%! This statistic truly is both shocking and sad. What percentage was your latest meal?

With a statistic such as this, who can be surprised at the state of health in this country? We are blindly, silently programming our DNA to trigger disease. It's heartbreaking when you really think about it. People simply don't know what they don't know.

Now, if you are someone who knows more about the science of food, then you realize that there is a lot more you can do to proactively stimulate positive epigenomic behavior within your body. Simply start avoiding those high sugar, empty-carb foods that make a negative impact on you—at both the DNA-cellular level as well as within your neural-synapse connections.

It's easy to fall into this trap—this type of food is the most readily available in our society. It's in every aisle of the grocery store. You have to read the label of most everything you eat to avoid it. And, it tastes good as well. Plus, it feels good (at first) to eat it. Crackers, bread, baked goods, sodas—these are our go-to comfort foods.

However, I tell my clients that every time they think of indulging in empty carbs such as donuts, cookies, and sodas (one of the worst offenders), to think of those carbs as "barbs," because they are literally splicing up your brain's superhighways by pulling calories from your brain cells and leaving them empty. This creates ragged, disjointed neural connections.

It also could be creating a plaque build-up around your neurons. This is a sticky protein that builds up around nerve cells, called amyloid plaque. It is toxic to neurons and could be the culprit behind memory loss. But what if this plaque build-up is a preventative mechanism? What if amyloid binding is actually hiding an infection underneath it? This could be one of the body's many self-defense mechanisms to protect itself from the toxic foods we eat.

The next Pillar is really two in one…

PILLARS 4 & 5: MOTION-EMOTION.

First, Motion. When our body is in motion, it triggers the release of several hormones and neurotransmitters, including insulin, glucagon, cortisol, epinephrine, norepinephrine, testosterone, human growth hormone, IGF, and BDNF (a neurotransmitter or nerve growth factor that stimulates the production of new cells in the brain and even within the digestive tract).

As professional athletes and bodybuilders know, there is a balance here. Too much exercise can trigger an unhealthy blend of chemicals. Too little doesn't provide the potential benefits. Again, each of these biological and chemical responses sends information to our epigenetic triggers that either opens up or diminishes health within our cells. And again, although the importance of movement and exercise in creating a healthy body has long been promoted, we have barely scratched the surface of how much this activity promotes health at the core of our being—that is, within our DNA.

And this just in: BDNF (brain-derived neurotrophic factor) is also wonderfully stimulated by exercise!

Moving your body is one of the single best ways you can boost neuron-synapses connections.

So, how much movement do you get in a day?

To promote brain health, make it a goal to get in some form of movement—biking, walking, running, or swimming—for at least 20 minutes twice per day. Think about how you can engage others in movement—can you walk with your spouse after dinner every night? Or play ball with your children or grandchildren? Consider how you can make movement a part of your everyday routine!

Then, Emotion. Our emotions are direct links to our hormones, and therefore direct triggers to our DNA functions. Crying carries stress hormones out of the body. Simply writing about a loved one can also reduce stress levels. The feeling of gratitude and contentment triggers the production of oxytocin, which increases the flow of oxygen to tissues and promotes harmonious electric activity around both your heart and brain. Falling in love can quicken the growth of our nerve cells for as much as a year. Laughter has been shown to boost beta-endorphins by 27%, as well as the human growth hormone by 87%.

In contrast, an argument with a loved one can reduce your body's ability to heal for at least a day. Even when you simply think about or recall an argument, it can raise blood pressure, heart rate, and adrenaline levels. Chronic stress—the mac-daddy of negative emotive triggers—cues adrenaline, as well as a host of other hormones, and in the process turns off long-term cellular building and repair projects. Stress has also been linked directly to many, many diseases. However, when we look at it from a deeper level, it's even scarier than we originally thought—because it turns off important parts of our DNA. Depression lowers the amount of serotonin, a neuron-growing hormone in our brains... which in turn, makes us more susceptible to physical aches, pains, and sadness.

ALL of this clearly illustrates that our emotions immediately trigger chemical and hormonal responses in our bodies, which in turn, trigger epigenetic cues that turn our DNA potential on or off.

Emotions can act in a nanosecond to stimulate both positive and negative reactions in our bodies. If your emotions have been predominately negative over the past week or more, look for new ways to create joy and gratitude in your life. It is not just for the sake of enjoying the day-to-day moments in your life; you are literally shaping the quality of your health and therefore, your future.

PILLAR 6: BREATH

Because it is such an integral part of our involuntary nervous system, we kind of take it for granted. The concept of water as a fundamental and important ingredient within our bodies has become more popularized and understood. However, air, the basic basis of life, is often overlooked.

Did you ever think about what happens to the oxygen you breathe?

On a regular basis, we don't think about the quality of the air we breathe, nor the quantity we train ourselves to take in with each breath. Breathing is so easy and common that we just do it, blindly. However, practicing deep breathing techniques and thereby training ourselves to breathe slower and more deeply, can have tremendous health benefits—in both the short- and long-term.

For one, breathing can quickly shift negative emotional states to more positive states. However, quality breathing also increases energy and provides deep nourishment to our cells. Yes, your red blood cells carry oxygen to each cell in your body, but then what? We breathe for our mitochondria, a tiny organelle within each cell that pushes power into your life in the form of energy. Mitochondria actually use your breath to create mito-respiration as part of a cycle to make energy, also known as ATP, within you. In fact, 90% of the oxygen coming into your cells is used to create the energy that fuels your entire body.

Most of my clients are shallow breathers and are thereby cheating their mitochondria the power they need to make more energy. And as a result of this energy loss, they are cheating themselves of their body's natural ability to turn on healthy genes.

PILLAR 7: SLEEP

Did you know that when you sleep you are basically "putting your body in the shop" to repair? When you sleep, your entire system detoxes and regenerates. Your brain clears out waste, which supports learning and memory. This process also helps us to regulate emotions and make positive decisions. In addition, as you sleep, proteins are regulated and put to use throughout your body. In laymen's terms, that means it is when your body repairs itself, gets rid of toxins, and builds new cells and tissues. In fact, just losing one night of sleep can change your genomic pillars for the worse. Scientifically speaking, it is the fastest known way to alter those DNA-Cellular-Mitochondrial-Neuronal-Synapse connections. All in all, if you do not sleep well or regularly, your body will not be able to get into a repair shop to fix itself. And you are quickly creating genomic triggers that will make you more susceptible to chronic illness; especially Alzheimer's disease, dementia, and cognitive disorders.

PILLAR 8: RESILIENCE

This is our ability to adapt and respond in spite of the adversities we face in life. It's our ability to turn "toxic stress" into "tolerable stress." This is a psychological stamina that we develop over time through both reactive and proactive conditioning. In short, it's the conversations we have with ourselves in our heads. Resilience is when we tell ourselves to move on, to find a better way, and to motivate positive change. It is the story we tell ourselves about who we are, and what is possible for us in the world.

From a scientific perspective, this sort of "self-talk" can make or break our cells. Essentially, when we can take a negative situation and turn it into something positive, we begin to navigate life's circumstances. We put ourselves in that coveted "driver's seat." From here, we can choose to change our life trajectory. This is the place where we set the rules; where nothing dictates what is possible—not parents, not teachers, not awful memories or situations, and not even the bill of health predicted by our doctors.

This ability changes the game—because it changes everything. It is the "it" factor that gives us the resolve to consciously and strategically shift every single other genomic pillar I've shared. Resilience is the bridge that connects the rest of the 7 genomic pillars. If we are predominately weak in most of these areas, our resilience is also weak. If we are predominately strong in each of the other pillars, our resilience will also be strong.

Most of my clients have at least 3-4 genomic pillars in chaos. Each of these genomic pillars is interconnected and therefore, improving one can lead to improvements in each of the others.

If you build up your resilience, it can create a strong surge of momentum that can turn absolutely everything around.

It is like a ripple that can extend out and positively impact the entire spectrum.

Our resilience in the face of what we currently know and understand is what *makes us human.* That drive is what has, over time, triggered our DNA to evolve and progress into this amazing, creative, beautiful force of life that we are today.

ONE FINAL MESSAGE

And so, my message for you is this—our future is bright.

We do not have to accept the limitations of the previously thought "incurable" diseases and conditions that we face as a human race.

Our only challenge is to understand how powerful we really are. And to thereby make decisions to aid our body in doing what it miraculously already knows how to do…

Research dictates that no one has ever recovered from Alzheimer's disease—UNTIL 2014, and with the science of epigenomics now we have hope. **There are almost 100 different "holes" or DNA-cellular-mitochondrial-neuron-synapses that have been dimmed and that we need to turn back on to reverse the disease.** However, our bodies are so brilliant that if we can just turn ten of them back on, the body will start to heal itself and begin turning the others on.

However, even more than treating this disease and other cognitive disorders, we need to prevent them. And we must start earlier and earlier. Currently, we see the beginning of cognitive decline show up most commonly in people in their 50s-60s who have been coping with a high-stress job for several years, as they simply start to "forget" things. However, in modern times, with so much processed food, an increased lack of exercise, and a poor diet, we are seeing signs of cognitive decline show up in people in their 40s and even mid-30s.

We need to wake up! We need to move this needle and to start making our health the priority. Because once it's gone, it is the *only* priority. The earlier we start, the better.

Pressure to change from a reactive medical state to proactive treatment and care will not happen until we demand this shift, together. We need to put the 'we' back in wellness. Families with this decline cannot do it alone. Together, we can focus the science more and more from cellular "illness" dynamics to cellular "wellness" dynamics.

Together, we can each apply and use these 8 pillars to reverse disease in those we love and to stimulate well-being in ourselves to avoid and eliminate these disorders altogether.

In the fight against disease—including Alzheimer's disease, dementia, and cognitive disorders—there is HOPE.

And it starts with you.

In closing this chapter, I'd like to share a poem, "The Impossible Dream." This is what inspires me to continue on this journey, facing challenges and uncertainty along the way. I hope that it will inspire you to do the same.

THE IMPOSSIBLE DREAM

To dream the impossible dream
To fight the unbeatable foe
To bear with unbearable sorrow
To run where the brave dare not go

To right the un-rightable wrong
To love pure and chaste from afar
To try when your arms are too weary
To reach the unreachable star

This is my quest to follow that star
No matter how hopeless, no matter how far
To fight for the right
Without question or pause
To be willing to march
Into hell for a heavenly cause.

Words: Joe Darion, Music: Mitch Leigh

CHAPTER TWO REFERENCES

Szalavitz, M. Touching Empathy: Lack of physical affection can actually kill babies; Psychology Today; https://www.psychologytoday.com/us/blog/born-love/201003/touching-empathy. Published March 1, 2010. Accessed February 2018.

Taylor, J. Personal Growth: Motivation: The drive to change. Do you have the drive to change your life? Psychology Today; https://www.psychologytoday.com/blog/the-power-prime/201201/personal-growth-motivation-the-drive-change. Published January 2, 2012. Accessed February 2018.

Stephens, A. The link between emotions and health. Psychologies; https://www.psychologies.co.uk/self/the-link-between-emotions-and-health.html. Published August 24, 2011. Accessed February 2018.

McCall, P. 8 hormones involved in exercise. American Council on Exercise; https://www.acefitness.org/blog/5593/8-hormones-involved-in-exercise. Published August 10, 2015. Accessed February 2018.

Weil, A. The art and science of breathing. Weil: Andrew Weil, MD; https://www.drweil.com/health-wellness/balanced-living/meditation-inspiration/the-art-and-science-of-breathing/. Accessed February 2018.

IFLScience. One night of sleep deprivation can affect the genes that control the biological clocks in your cells. IFLScience; http://www.iflscience.com/health-and-medicine/one-night-sleep-deprivation-can-affect-genes-control-biological-clocks-your/. Accessed February 2018.

Peever J, Murray, BJ. What happens in the brain during sleep? Scientific American; https://www.scientificamerican.com/article/what-happens-in-the-brain-during-sleep1/. Accessed February 2018.

Walsh, B. The science of resilience: why some children can thrive despite adversity. Harvard Graduate School of Education; https://www.gse.harvard.edu/news/uk/15/03/science-resilience. Published March 23, 2015. Accessed February 2018.

Johnson AL. The DNA of Hope. Christiana, PA. Ann-Louise Johnson, 2018.

Gómez-Pinilla F. Brain foods: the effects of nutrients on brain function. Nature reviews Neuroscience. 2008;9(7):568-578. doi:10.1038/nrn2421.

Simpson NS, Scott-Sutherland J, Gautam S, Sethna N, Haack M. Chronic exposure to insufficient sleep alters processes of pain habituation and sensitization. Pain. 2018 Jan; 159(1): 33-40.

Ngandu T, Lehtisalo J, Solomon A, et al. A 2 year multidomain intervention of diet, exercise, cognitive training, and vascular risk monitoring versus control to prevent cognitive decline in at-risk elderly people (FINGER): a randomised controlled trial. Lancet. 2015 June 6; 385:2255–63.

Ryan KK, Seeley RJ. Food as a Hormone. Science (New York, NY). 2013; 339(6122): 918-919. doi:10.1126/science.1234062.

Tononi G, Massimini M, Riedner BA. Sleepy dialogues between cortex and hippocampus: who talks to whom? Neuron. 2006 Dec 7; 52(5): 748-9. https://doi.org/10.1016/j.neuron.2006.11.014.

Moorcroft TA. Physiology and Biochemistry of Mindfulness, Sleep, and Exercise. Origins of Health website. www.originsofhealth.com.

Bredesen DE, Amos EC, Canick J, et al. Reversal of cognitive decline in Alzheimer's disease. Aging (Albany NY). 2016; 8(6):1250-1258. doi:10.18632/aging.100981.

THE 8 SENSES: YOUR SECRET LIFELINE WEAPON

Operation Hope is all about providing enthusiastic support for your team, and support for every cell and its performance or metabolism within you.

Metabolism = Your cell power within you to strengthen and repair you.

Today, you're going to uncover a lifeline, a secret weapon to rescue, save, and pull yourself and the ones you love out of danger.

In cognitive decline, you want to slow down, repair, and reverse the damage by growing new brain cells and neurons.

HOW IS YOUR LIFELINE?

What is your support? How strong is it? Is your lifeline powered up? Are you able to slow down, repair, and reverse damage and grow new neurons and brain cells within you? Are you boosting your own performance? Is your lifeline restoring hope?

Until 2014, no lifeline existed for Alzheimer's. No one lived, no one came back to his or her family or workplace. No one! Now we can! Because we have HOPE.

THREE PRINCIPLES OF LIFELINES

1: **This Lifeline is a very special LIFE-line that can bring you back.** It rekindles life and health. Also: It can bring you back to what you were… and perhaps even more!

2: **A secretly coded Lifeline mobilizes support**—such as outside support groups and inside support molecules. Your Lifeline is coded with secret codes that support healing for a more vibrant life and health.

3: **It takes a hero to learn how to use this secret Lifeline.** With some training and true enthusiasm, a hero can revive hope using this Lifeline.

The first Lifeline is right inside of you or your loved one: The 8 Senses Lifeline. Our senses are like a key that unlocks unused brain areas and awakens repair and healing powers within us. They turn nerve cells, or neurons, into a molecular gym inside of us.

Neuron: a specialized cell transmitting nerve impulses; a nerve cell.

Your neurons are the key players in your brain. They are at work right now as you read this. Neurons are information messengers. By way of example, imagine driving down the highway for 500 miles towards a city you've never visited. But there's a problem with your trip. There are no signs, no stop lights, no nighttime highway lighting, no names of states or cities on billboards, and no exit numbers. How would you know where you were going? You wouldn't. Now add neurons to your trip. Everything lights up. Through electrical impulses, your brain's neurons give you information and direction. Neurons are the conduit between your brain and the rest of your nervous system. It is impossible to read, think, or feel without them. They tell you where to go and how to get there.

You can coach, motivate, support, feed, and strengthen nerves—your neurons.

Now grab onto that Lifeline and mobilize it to become a HERO as both of you, together, rescue these 8 Senses.

This takes enthusiasm. This takes knowledge, power, and training.

H.O.P.E. = H.eroes O.perating with P.ower and E.nthusiasm

It's time to restore, reboot, and rescue HOPE of growing new neurons now by mobilizing the Lifeline of the 8 Senses.

SENSE 1: TOUCH

Touch is the ability to feel something—really feel it.

"Our tactile world is rich, if not infinite. The flutter of an insect's wings, a warm breeze, a blunt object, raindrops, and a mother's gentle caress impose mechanical forces upon the skin, and yet we encounter no difficulty in telling them apart and react differently to each. How do we recognize and interpret the myriad of tactile stimuli to perceive the richness of the physical world? Aristotle classified touch, along with vision, hearing, smell, and taste, as one of the five main senses."

—The Sensory Neurons of Touch, by
Victoria E. Abraira and David D. Ginty

When you truly touch, you feel it so much, it is almost as if you can taste it. True touch encompasses all in such a way that you can hear it, taste it, smell it… with your hands, underneath your feet, against your face. When you touch, you are able to sense when it is hot or cold; you are able to feel when something is sharp versus smooth, or sticky versus slick.

However, for those experiencing cognitive decline, the sense of touch is decreased. Therefore, patients with cognitive disorders such as Alzheimer's have the potential to injure themselves more easily if they were to touch a hot stove or step on something sharp.

But touch can also be one of the most effective ways to start bringing back your brain cells and neurons.

By focusing on the power of touch, your touch neurons—which are some of the fastest in the human body—you can increase your ability, or that of your loved one, to begin to feel presence more readily again. So, set out daily to intentionally activate and engage with your sense of touch. Hold your partner's hand. Reach out to your friends and family every time you greet them, engaging your sense of touch. Maybe lay your hand on their shoulder, offer a hug or a gentle nudge. Let your neurons remember how to feel again by experiencing touch.

As caregivers and support-team members, your own interactions with your loved ones can help immensely in engaging their sense of touch. So you, too, touch and caress and help your loved one connect with the world around them through their sense of touch.

SENSE 2: TASTE

Taste is our ability to perceive or experience the flavor of something.

Without taste, life is extremely dull. Taste allows us to perceive one of the greatest joys—food! Being able to taste food also allows us to re-experience moments and people in our lives.

From a practical standpoint, life without the taste sense can be dangerous. If, for example, someone cannot tell the difference between salt and sugar. Or soap and sugar. Being such an integral part of how our bodies work, when younger people lose their taste, it alerts us to possible early symptoms of cognitive decline. Taste and smell are often the first senses to disappear. So, this is a good way to test someone's cognitive state.

Did you know that our sense of taste is dependent on having key minerals in your system?

So, make sure you are, or your patient is, on a good, absorbable, multivitamin.

Also, do not let cognitive decline keep you from experimenting with flavors—spices, textures, mixtures, and combinations of different foods. Try foods you've known forever, that take you back to when you were small and ran around the yard as your family celebrated holidays. Eat food you've never tasted before, that will excite your taste buds and awaken your sense of taste.

SENSE 3: SMELL

Smell is the capacity to perceive or detect the odor or scent of something.

As mentioned before, **smell is a partner sense to taste,** and it is often the first sense to decline with cognitive disorders.

The great thing about your sense of smell is that we can use the nuances of smell to both test and reawaken the senses. For example, often in support groups, we will ask:

"Can you smell cinnamon?" "Can you smell the difference between cinnamon and mint?" And then, "Can you smell with BOTH sides of the nose?"

As with the sense of touch, losing the sense of smell can be dangerous. For example, if there is a gas leak in the house and you are unable to identify the situation by the smell of gas. Also, even the inability to smell food can be hazardous to one's health. As you know, smell stimulates appetite. So, not having a sense of smell could possibly trigger bad food choices, or sometimes eliminate appetite completely. Thus, it is common to find significant weight loss issues with the loss of the sense of smell.

As a way to maintain the sense of smell, cook more and refrigerate less.

This may sound radical in our society; however, there is sound science behind it. When our body is not operating at its best, it becomes more sensitive to food allergies—it becomes a histamine issue. Refrigerated foods, especially, grow more histamine, which is what triggers food allergies and food sensitivities in the first place.

When your body desperately needs the rich nutrients in natural food to heal itself, you don't want to stress the process by making your body fight *against* the food you are eating.

Now, to open new brain pathways, we can smell different scents: spices, flowers, objects, and things the person loves—even the scented shirt of a loved one. By smelling specific scents the person has strong affectionate links to, you are able to help reawaken memories, which in turn are strongly linked to emotions. As you stimulate this entire pathway of neural connections, you trigger the molecules that can brighten DNA's function and kick-start healing.

SENSE 4: SIGHT

The ability to see—color, rainbows, clouds, nature.

Seeing is visual stimulation—reading, gazing at inspiring scenery, and seeing the faces of family members and people they recognize can all stimulate a person's sense of sight.

Losing sight makes it easier for people to fall, so for this reason, one of the best things you can do for someone whose sight has declined is to remove anything they can trip on—throw rugs, loose stuff in walkways, etc. So often this simple tip is forgotten, leading to hip or arm fractures.

It is also common for individuals with cognitive decline to lose the ability to recognize shapes and faces. **But, can we awaken these sleeping brain areas? We can try because Together We Can!**

Remember: It takes a Hero, and it takes a Lifeline.

You can use the sense of sight as a Lifeline to reawaken very specific brain areas. Taking your loved one or patient anyplace that is visually stimulating will help. However, if you do take a patient outside, **make sure they have sunglasses on**, so that it's not over-stimulating. **You want them to be able to look around peacefully and pleasantly**, not squinting or shading their eyes the entire time.

Another great way to stimulate the sense of sight is having their main rooms and living areas be colorful, bright, and upbeat.

Finally, **reading is a great way to reawaken the sense of sight**. If you worry about those who can no longer hold a book or focus on the words, you can find amazing books in audiobook format. Because audiobooks evoke words—words they've interacted with via their sense of sight for so long—you are able to stimulate the brain and restart neuron growth.

For each of these senses, our ultimate goal is to wake up the brain and help nerve connections grow new pathways. So: go gently, go slow, but start! GO NOW! You are the Hero here!

SENSE 5: HEARING

Hearing is the ability to perceive sounds.

Hearing is a key element of memory stimulation. I call it hippo-memory because it is part of the hippocampus's memory pathway.

This means that when people have a good sense of hearing, they:

1. Have a better memory
2. Learn more easily
3. Have a good sense of space and balance

These are all things our brain's hippocampus helps us with.

Some people have a keener sense of hearing than others. Unfortunately, the stronger our sense of hearing is to start, the more it can throw us off when it is diminished. A diminished sense of hearing can actually make you feel quite isolated and confined. As you lose your hearing, it can feel as if you are in a cave.

In working with people who have a cognitive disorder, you want to **avoid loud noises that could startle or disorient them**. Instead, you want to approach them slowly, and then offer up a touch so that they know you're there. And then, speak gently to them, in a tone that doesn't feel invasive or too strong.

And here is another secret:

If you have lost any of these senses, **start using them**.

Start kicking in that memory of smells, of images, of tastes… That's right, do what you can't, so you can again!

You read correctly: Do what you can't… so you can again!

SENSE 6: PROPRIOCEPTION

Proprioception is the perception or awareness of the position of one's body.

The sense of proprioception is new to many people. It is a combination of many of our senses, and it defines your place in space. It's a sort of **body self-awareness**. Are you standing straight? Are you sitting straight? Are you balanced enough to walk without falling? Can you perceive the difference between an uphill slope and a downhill slope?

These are important senses. For Parkinson's patients, this is one of the major senses they struggle with. They're especially at risk of falling backward. Therefore, you always want to be concerned with safety.

One of the best techniques to use in re-awakening the sense of proprioception is to walk with someone. And if you are worried about their lack of stability, you can use what's known as a **"walking belt."**

A walking belt is a thick belt that someone can wear, with essentially a handle in the back that you can use to provide extra support and/or to catch them in case of a fall.

Work with a therapist or someone who knows how to use a walking belt. It's a great safe mobility tool!

Proprioception can also be awakened by any type of exercise, physical motion, or strength training. Increased physical activity can especially help people with Alzheimer's and Parkinson's.

About 25 years ago, I was the lead in creating a senior exercise and vitality center, which focused on using exercise as a way to rehabilitate seniors ages 55 to 90.

Throughout my time there, I witnessed countless cases of people who went from shaking so badly they couldn't even hold an object, to having strong, steady muscles and being able to get out of a chair without using their arms. It was amazing to see how so many **men and women were reclaiming their independence and happiness through consistent, regular exercise**.

In addition, through this center, we also scientifically studied how exercise makes a person feel better, emotionally and physically. The results indicated that the more exercise an individual did, the more independent they felt, and thus, the less healthcare utilization was needed—meaning **people were using fewer medications, requiring fewer hospitalizations, staying healthier, and feeling better**. They had more LIFE and more enjoyable time with their social group.

That is why exercise can make a real impact!

And I want to emphasize—

You are never too old to move and begin strength training and exercising.

People with cognitive disorders often suffer from sarcopenia, or weak muscles, and much of this is from lack of use. So, let's use these muscles; it's time to move more to be more!

Never think life is over if you have weak muscles. Unfortunately, this is what people with declining health often think. But we can change that way of thinking together. Regarding muscles and strength: use it or lose it! **But, as I always recommend, it's better to never lose it! Move more!**

For example, I have a friend who has Parkinson's, and for 15 years, he wouldn't engage in any type of exercise. Recently, we got him on a bike—it took three people to help him to get on the bike initially—that's correct, three people—but now he spends about 17 minutes on it every day! And he has gone from freezing up every couple of minutes to quite literally running down the halls.

SENSE 7: TO REMEMBER

To Remember: The ability to access our precious, beautiful memories.

Both long- and short-term memory are critical. However, for this segment, I am focusing on short-term memory.

To remember is your ability to recall dates, your daily calendar, what's on your schedule for the next day, when to take a certain medication, when to eat, etc.

I am focusing on this type of memory here because lack of it is one of the key factors leading to a feeling of isolation.

As patients, again and again, forget the little details, their families begin to lose touch with them, which can create a downward spiral.

SENSE 8: SUPPORT

Support is the feeling of togetherness.

Our last and eighth sense is support.

The 8 Senses together bring people together. **All of our senses bring our entire body within us together** which creates our sense of support, or togetherness.

Togetherness is an experience we share as humans, and the sense of support is at the heart of the Hope message. Because cognitive disorders have been traditionally labeled as "hopeless" and "incurable," many people give up on themselves and on loved ones suffering from such disorders.

Many people often think there is no way to get their loved one "back"… no way to get their mom, their dad, their grandparent or friend back.

But that is not the truth! Remember:

I CAN!

You CAN support your parent or loved one. You CAN give your loved ones tools to remember. You can AWAKEN those senses that trigger deep cellular and genetic responses within them—and within yourself.

You can begin to reverse their symptoms and trigger healing. Be a HERO and start helping someone!

Revive H.O.P.E.

So many of my patients before coming to us have lost their support group, which is a critical part of healing.

Having a group of people—friends and/or family—**who believe in them and who believe they will recover is the most powerful stimulant for healing**.

The reality for Alzheimer's, dementia, and cognitive decline is that it is a family affair.

Family and friend support is the denominator in reversing these brain challenges.

Make it a family affair.

Simply knowing that someone will support a patient in any way possible will keep that person motivated to reach for a higher level of health and wellness.

CHAPTER THREE REFERENCES

Valentin LSS. Can Digital Games Be a Way of Improving the Neuroplasticity in Stroke Damage? Can the Adult Brain Grow New Cells or Rewire Itself in Response to a New Experience? Open Journal of Medical Psychology. 2017 Apr 8; 6:153-165. doi: 10.4236/ojmp.2017.62013.

Lledo PM, Valley M. Adult Olfactory Bulb Neurogenesis.Cold Springs Harbor Perspectives in Biology. 2016, May 27; 8(8): pii: a018945. doi: 10.1101/cshperspect.a018945.

Monti DA, Zabrecky G, Kremens D, et al. N-Acetyl Cysteine May Support Dopamine Neurons in Parkinson's Disease: Preliminary Clinical and Cell Line Data. Wang Y, ed. PLoS ONE. 2016;11(6):e0157602. doi:10.1371/journal.pone.0157602.

Stangl D, Thuret S. Impact of diet on adult hippocampal neurogenesis. Genes & Nutrition. 2009; 4(4): 271-282. doi:10.1007/s12263-009-0134-5.

Oka Y, Katada S, Omura M, Suwa M, Yoshihara Y, Touhara K. Odorant Receptor Map in the Mouse Olfactory Bulb: In Vivo Sensitivity and Specificity of Receptor-Defined Glomeruli. Neuron. 2009 Dec 7; 52:857–869.

Fjaeldstad A, Fernandes HM, Van Hartevelt TJ, et al. Brain fingerprints of olfaction: a novel structural method for assessing olfactory cortical networks in health and disease. Sci. Rep. 2017 Feb 14; 7:42534.

Abraira VE, Ginty DD. The Sensory Neurons of Touch. Neuron. 2013; 79(4):10.1016/j.neuron.2013.07.051. doi:10.1016/j.neuron.2013.07.051.

Selkoe DJ. Alzheimer's Disease Is a Synaptic Failure. Science. 2002 Oct 25; 298:789-791. doi: 10.1126/science.1074069.

CHAPTER FOUR
YOUR TREASURE M.A.P.

W here in the world do we see more enthusiasm than at a circus?

Remember the circus: the music, the colors, the laughter! The performers, the animals, popcorn, and cotton candy. And of course, the clowns. Do you remember the high wire walkers?

As a kid, I always wondered: How do they find the courage to balance way up high, on just a tiny wire? Just watching that daring feat brought my heart rate up and made me sweat.

Today, I would like to share a story with you about a client who was a high wire artist. As I go through his story, I will be creating a M.A.P.—clues to use to find hidden health concerns.

Now, I introduce you to Perry P. Perrington.

Perry was a daring highwire walker who performed flawlessly for years, until one day he fell off the wire. When I first met Perry, he was furious. Injured and defeated, his courage was replaced with an overwhelming rage and he revealed in his eyes a constant undercurrent of raw fear.

I share this story about Perry with you because Perry was a sort of Alzheimer's "perfect storm." What I mean by this is that **there are certain ingredients that set the stage for the onset of cognitive decline**. These ingredients could have remained hidden in the past, **but today, you are there—watching this brain-drama unfold**.

With Perry—as with many—I could see it coming from miles away. But the sooner we are able to understand how these ingredients affect our cognitive health, the sooner we can work to change things. Why? Because…

Lifestyle changes are the key to success in getting your memory and brain back.

REVIEW: THE 8 GENOMIC PILLARS

As a reminder, your health relies on 8 core pillars that build and support wellness and vitality or illness and decline. I call these pillars the 8 Genomic Pillars, and they are:

1. Support

2. Motivation

3. Food

4. Motion

5. Emotion

6. Breath

7. Sleep

8. Resilience

The 8 Genomic Pillars can make or break your health trajectory and it is imperative that you understand how they do so, because the way they work is the high wire walk you take daily at home, work, and everywhere you go.

Any time we travel somewhere new, the best way to get there is with the assistance and direction provided by a map. That is why, to help you answer the question of whether you are, or your loved one is, a perfect storm, I'm sharing with you a M.A.P. for cognitive vitality. As you journey into this new land of self-discovery, look to this M.A.P. to lead the way.

M.A.P.

M.A.P. is an acronym that stands for Measure, Aim, and Pace.

Measure is the **ability to know where you are right now**. Using simple tests, tools, and techniques that I will share with you, you'll be able to figure out where you are right now, within each of these pillars.

Aim is **the direction in which you are heading**. It's where you want to go. You could call this a "goal," however, the word "aim" feels more accurate to me, because the moment you take action to make positive, healing changes in your life, is the moment you are already on the path and moving in a different direction. Also, the word AIM in itself functions as the acronym A.I.M., where you can **Assess** the situation, **Implement** new changes, and then continually **Measure** them to redirect and focus your energy, as needed.

Pace is about **knowing how you are moving on the path**. How many positive new behaviors are you taking on this fight *for* healing and wellness against disease? Are you getting rid of toxicity? Are you integrating new commitments and life changes? Are you working to reverse cognitive decline, or practicing avoidance?

Within this M.A.P you find these 8 Genomic Pillars—but within each of these Pillars are 3 levels or 3 dimensions, like a 3D model, and they are: Structure, Function, and Behavior.

Within every living and non-living object, there is a Structure, Function, and Behavior. Each of these layers is linked, impacting the next layer. A specific **Structure** will have a specific **Function**, which ultimately will have a very specific **Behavior**.

Structure gives us the geography of our problem, Function provides the mechanics, and Behavior gives us the topography or the practical view of our challenge face-to-face.

So, on our M.A.P. for cognitive vitality as it relates to health, the three core layers of Structure, Function, and Behavior can be understood as three core dimensions:

1. Health Blueprint (Structure)

2. Cellular Blueprint (Function)

3. DNA and Genes Blueprint (Behavior)

1. HEALTH BLUEPRINT (STRUCTURE)

Your Health Blueprint **is your physical structure, and it includes the habits, environments, illnesses, stressors, etc. that are either helping or hindering your daily performance.** The 8 Genomic Pillars are part of this Health Blueprint layer.

Think of this layer as **the story of how and why you got here in your health or illness**—your personal health journey from pre-birth, birth, and all the way to this moment in time. Everything in this timeline affects you today, including *how* you were born, be it natural birth or C-section.

For example, a child born by C-Section would have been exposed to different types of bacteria or microbes from the mother than during a traditional birth. This could lead to more health problems in the child as he or she gets older, like more allergies and sensitivities that could alter this person's health throughout life!

How? Well, a baby's immune cells are "trained"—so to speak—by the **structure** of the microbes they meet. Birth canal microbes train one way. The skin's microbes train another way—and these are the microbes a baby born by C-section receives.

Your Health Blueprint, your health story, MATTERS, including your birth story…

2. CELLULAR BLUEPRINT (FUNCTION)

The middle Functional layer in the M.A.P. is the Cellular Blueprint.

Cells are all about function, and they tell us how your body is functioning deep inside. When you go for an annual physical and your doctor asks you to get blood work, he or she is doing so in order to evaluate your health at this cellular layer.

For example, at the cellular layer, you could see if your protein levels are normal, high or low, or somewhere in between. **A functional understanding of your cells can provide a lot of information about how food is absorbed and utilized deep within each cell**.

As you change your Health Blueprint by micro or macro changes in any of the 8 Genomic Pillars—food, relationships, sleep, etc.—we can actually see and measure very specific changes at the molecular cellular layer.

3. DNA AND GENES BLUEPRINT (BEHAVIOR)

The deepest layer of our M.A.P. for cognitive vitality is called your DNA and Genes Blueprint. **Your DNA and your genes establish and determine how your body behaves, repairs, makes new cells, and more**. This deepest layer is in constant communication with the other layers, directing everything that happens within your body.

At the DNA and Genes Blueprint layer, we can see what Single Nucleotide Polymorphisms (or SNPs, read "snips") you have. What does SNPs mean? **A SNP is a gene mutation**. We all have a lot of them, but what matters is *where* you have them as well as *how much* the SNP's behavior affects your body's structure and function.

For efficiency and simplicity's sake, I often suggest to my clients that genes typically operate at 100%, 60%, or 10%. A 10% functioning gene occurs when you receive a SNP from both parents. However, this does not mean you can't overcome this disadvantage.

If you have a lesser functioning gene, you may just need to take in extra nutrients so they can surround that gene and help it to properly express at the cellular layer.

How can you set yourself and your brain up to win? Create your M.A.P. Your M.A.P. will be your Treasure Map; it will allow you to measure where you are, aim into a new direction—the direction of healing and newness—learn more, be more, do more, and share more…. Oh, the treasures you will find!

So, set a pace to move yourself forward, **one step at a time**, with enthusiasm and motivation.

Your brain is waiting for you.

CHAPTER FOUR REFERENCES

Hellmann DB, Ziegelstein RC. Personomics: A New Series in the Green Journal. American Journal of Medicine . 2017 June; 130(6):622.

Matias Rodrigues JF, Wagner A. Evolutionary Plasticity and Innovations in Complex Metabolic Reaction Networks. PLoS Computational Biology. 2009 Dec 19; 5(12):e1000613.

Stilling RM, Dinan TG, Cryan JF. The brain's Geppetto—microbes as puppeteers of neural function and behaviour? Journal of NeuroVirology. 2016 Feb 22; 22(1):14-21.

Alderton WK, Cooper CE, Knowles RG. Nitric oxide synthases: structure, function and inhibition. Biochem J. 2001 Aug 1; 357(Pt 3): 593-615.

Picciotto MR, Higley MJ, Mineur YS. Acetylcholine as a neuromodulator: cholinergic signaling shapes nervous system function and behavior. Neuron. 2012;76(1):116-129. doi:10.1016/j. neuron.2012.08.036.

Wagner A. How the global structure of protein interaction networks evolves. Proceedings of the Royal Society B: Biological Sciences. 2003;270(1514):457-466. doi:10.1098/rspb.2002.2269.

Wagner A, Fell DA. The small world inside large metabolic networks. Proceedings of the Royal Society B: Biological Sciences. 2001; 268(1478):1803-1810. doi:10.1098/rspb.2001.1711.

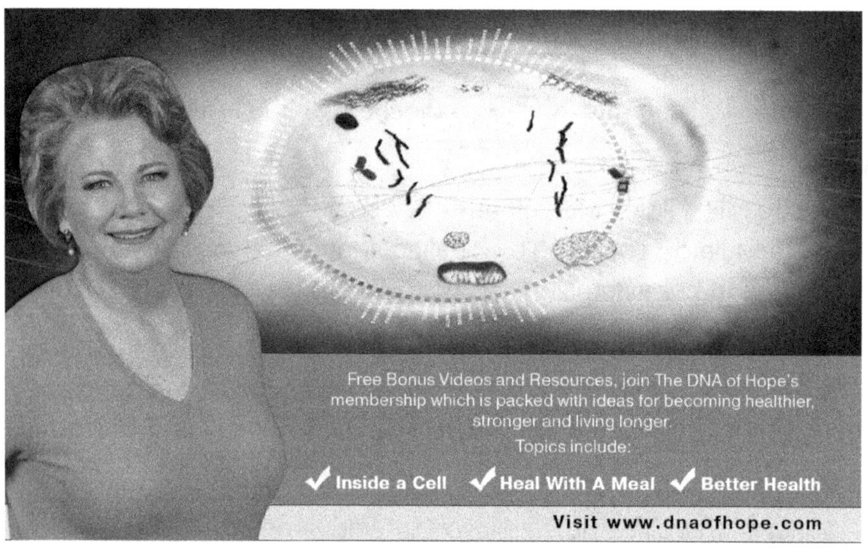
Free Bonus Videos and Resources, join The DNA of Hope's
membership which is packed with ideas for becoming healthier,
stronger and living longer.
Topics include:
Inside a Cell   Heal With A Meal   Better Health
Visit www.dnaofhope.com

A DIAGNOSIS OR PERSONALIZED MEDICINE

T he prevalent diagnoses of Alzheimer's, dementia, and cognitive decline in our world today is staggering. Yet, if there is life and breath, I promise—there is hope.

There is still hope.

In fact, let's take a step back and look at how these diseases are currently being diagnosed in the first place.

From a medical community perspective, we are currently operating somewhere between the 20th and 21st century. Most medical practitioners are beginning (albeit slowly) to think differently about how we diagnose and treat disease.

20th century thinking believes that "one size fits all" as far as treating disease goes. They identify what they believe a patient is suffering from, prescribe medication to treat that condition, and monitor the results. If the condition does not improve, they prescribe more medication. And if those medications create side effects that result in new conditions, they refer the patient to a "specialist" who can work on treating those conditions, most likely by prescribing more medications.

This line of thinking has been our medical mode of operation for over two decades. From 1984-2011, there have been no real changes in terms of how mainstream medicine diagnoses and treats disease. And for patients facing Alzheimer's, dementia, and cognitive decline, the diagnosis is basically a dead-end road. **Conventional 20th century medicine does not believe in a cure for this disease, and the only thing that they do offer is medication**. However, the medications they have given patients have not given them back their memory. They have not granted them the ability to go back to work. They haven't helped them enjoy positive, healing relationships again; or enjoy shopping, cooking, or going out to dinner; or brought them back to participating in their favorite hobbies, sports, or exercises.

There is no doubt—medications have failed us, especially in the realm of cognitive decline.

And with this insight, we have to realize—**we have been looking for a cure in the wrong place.**

Many reputable and respected physicians and medical practitioners of the 21st century have begun to turn the dial. **21st century medicine could be best described as "functional medicine."**

Rather than starting with the diagnosis, we start with the years leading up to the onset of disease, and we broaden our search to examine a much larger range of contributing factors that could be creating a patient's "perfect storm," including toxins, infections, lack of nutrients, hormone levels, melatonin levels, sleep deprivation, emotions, breath, and genomics.

21st century medicine believes that disease exists on spectrums and that there is a range of symptoms for disease… that show up differently for different people. We believe in personalized medicine, and personalized treatments specific to the unique make-up and history of each patient. We know that there is no "one-size-fits-all" wonder drug or treatment because every person is unique in Structure, Function, and Behavior.

In short, **a 21st century practitioner is constantly looking for the unique, individualized, root cause or causes of one's condition**—not at the variable symptoms that result because of that root.

Using this perspective and looking specifically at Alzheimer's, dementia, and cognitive decline, we have discovered that **there are currently only approximately 100 modifiers (or contributing factors) that can trigger these diseases**. Researchers in this field are currently still finalizing this number, but all agree, it's somewhere in this ballpark. Again, contributing factors are things like lack of sleep, lack of nutrition, hormone imbalance, poor GI health, lack of brain stimulation, lack of exercise, stress, etc.

In short:

There is a clear link between cognitive decline and the actions we take every day, as well as the environment we expose ourselves to—knowingly or unknowingly.

One of the most prominent researchers in this area, Dr. Dale Bredesen, describes these modifiers as "holes in your roof."— "The more you fix," Dr. Bredesen explains, "the less the roof will leak." However, we have found that **if you even just get 10 modifiers back in balance, the body's intelligence will kick in and actually work to fix the rest**—which is pretty extraordinary.

With this approach, **patients are not just living; they are thriving**. We have successfully returned memory performance and reversed cognitive decline. With regained function and as the memory returns, relationships have been restored and patients have regained their independence. They have returned to work, are driving again, and have ultimately been able to take care of their restored selves. In fact, **80% of patients overall with cognitive decline are now recovering!**

If you are currently fighting this battle, keep in mind—**the change happens gradually**. The first sign of improvement is that you simply stop declining. The second sign (which is bigger than we often acknowledge) is that you see any small sign of improvement. Think of it as a large ship that requires a lot of energy and momentum to turn. Even a small improvement is an indication that your ship has made the turn and is now moving in a positive, healing direction.

This chapter is definitely where things are starting to get exciting—we are really getting into the meat of how all of this comes together, as well as **what you can specifically do to reverse and/or prevent cognitive decline.**

In fact, there are a number of additional simple tests (many that I will share with you today) to help you determine your brain's current level of both speed and accuracy.

My goal is to inspire you to get curious. I want you to start to become a detective in your own life and to start looking for clues that may influence your cognitive health, long-term. I want you to want to look "underneath the hood." **I want to provide tools you can use to evaluate your current condition so that you can be more aware of exactly all of the contributing factors (or modifiers) that play a part in your own dynamic web of health**. We can now see changes in cell structure, function, and behavior long before a formal diagnosis is made, which gives us great headway in combatting all forms of cognitive decline.

HEALTH BLUEPRINT

As mentioned in the last chapter, this is your timeline, from birth to the current moment. And if you are currently working to improve your brain function, you should be constantly adding to this. **This is your personal pathway to healing and reversal, and with this in hand, if you do start to experience cognitive decline (and/or if you are already experiencing it at some level), you will be well equipped to provide this information to your doctor or medical practitioner**—which will save you critical time in terms of how you are treated. To some extent, you may also be able to begin healing yourself.

Most of my clients have no idea at first what could be causing their symptoms. Even after hours of interviews, they may still have no idea. For example, I recently interviewed a client for about an hour and a half, and we still couldn't figure it out. She finally admitted that it all seemed to start after she lost a significant amount of weight—which then easily clicked for me. Rapid weight loss will also result in a rapid release of toxins, which can overload the system.

EVOKE NEUROSCIENCE TEST

A second tool I want to share with you is a test that **can measure the speed and accuracy of your brain**—which is incredible. This is called the **Evoke Neuroscience Test**. This test **measures the electrical activity in the brain in response to the stimulation of specific sensory nerve pathways**. In essence, the test can pick up on cognitive changes in relation to both speed and accuracy that are too subtle to be noticed during a neurologic examination. You can take a test like this by visiting a practitioner, like me, who has this equipment.

This **brain map** is made to be about the size of a human brain. There is a front and back, right and left side, as labeled. Now I will label these areas and as I do, touch your brain area and then say it out loud—many of these words may be "first timers" for you, so say it out loud and start to get familiar with these parts of YOU.

Right now, we just want to get familiar with these areas. You don't need to spell them or memorize them. Each one of these structure areas has more functions than we can count. And each of these areas can cause quite specific symptoms when they get hurt—for instance, if they don't get enough food or circulation, or are injured in a fall, etc. A brain that is hurting can cause symptoms, and these symptoms can be precisely located to specific brain structure areas.

In a normal brain, you can notice the tight structure with very little space between the clefts, or fissures, as we call them. This is a younger brain, a thinking brain that has had exercise and lots of brain food and healthy fats— some things that keep a brain young. In the aging brain, you can see the fissures are wider and the structure looks weak and wrinkled. Also, the brain is smaller!

Some people shrink in height as they age, but did you know that the brain can shrink in size, too? It can, and we can measure it. However, **we can also reverse this condition**. We can grow our brain to increase its size (and power), but it takes a lot of dedication.

One of the fastest ways to increase your brain size is movement. Simply moving more or just walking more will make a difference. Eating healthy green, red, or purple vegetables helps, too.

With the healthy synapse, there is less space and a stronger signal. With the unhealthy synapse, there is more space between the neurons, which means a wider synapse and a longer area to push a signal. Just like a cell phone tower, distance matters; the longer the distance from cell towers (a.k.a. the neuron), the weaker the signal.

So, for example, if someone has a stroke, and is in a wheelchair, he or she must use whatever movement they can, such as in his or her arms—in order to keep his or her synapses firing. Or if a person is sensitive to smell, this person should insist on slowly re-introducing scents, with something like small doses of essential oils. In fact, just allowing a single drop of an essential oil in a glass of water placed in a nearby room would be beneficial for someone in this condition. You can see all of this on an Evoke Neuroscience Test.

OTHER TOOLS AND RESOURCES

There are also several tests and exercises you can do at home to test yourself. I would like to share some of them with you.

Waving Hands Exercise

This is a simple hand exercise that you can do yourself at home. Here's how it works. Stretch out your arms and hold your hands out in front of you, and wave them as fast as you can. Keep doing this for about a minute or two, then, start to notice if there is a difference in the speed of your hands, or in both hands. Can you move your fingers on both hands at the same speed? Is one hand moving slower than the other? As you continue to do this, does one hand fatigue faster?

Now rest your hands. This is a simple neurological test that you can do anytime. And I encourage you to test yourself this way, especially before and after incorporating new positive changes to any of your modifiers, such as getting more sleep, eating higher quality nutrients, etc.

Cell Phone Response Test

A simple test to try is to consider how well your cell phone responds to you. This sounds a bit crazy, but a touch-screen phone actually works not exactly from touch, but rather from the electro-conductivity produced by your touch. So, if key minerals are out of balance in your system, it may also feel like your phone "doesn't listen to you."

This is something I encourage you to try as homework following this module.

Additional At-Home Tests

The next couple of tests I'm sharing are also simple things you can do on your own. Remember Perry? This is a test I did with him. When he first came into my office, I asked Perry to **subtract 7 from 100**, and then to keep going. Perry's first answer was 77—and that's when I knew for sure that we were in trouble.

You see, **toxic metals in the system inhibit a person's ability to innumerate backward**. As you may recall, Perry suffered from a significant lack of nutrition. He was eating far more carbohydrates than proteins, and he was very low on quality fats.

Another quick test we did was to look at his fingernails and face. The lines in your fingernails are highly suggestive of low protein absorption. Rosacea, with those multiple broken blood vessels in your cheeks, can indicate low hydrochloric acid. The body needs hydrochloric acid for protein absorption.

Check out your fingernails. They provide a 6-month history of the nutrients in your system. You want to feel whether your nails are rough to touch and whether there are deep lines on your nails. This is a sign of poor protein absorption.

You too can heal, not tomorrow or next year, but starting today!

Remember—together we can dream the impossible dream.

Together we can fight that unbeatable foe.

Yes, together we can bear with unbearable sorrow that shattering diagnosis and then… **We are going to run where the brave dare not go**.

To shatter this diagnosis, we must run, not walk, where the brave dare not go… further, deeper, into the cellular, molecular, and genomic life deep inside of you, deeper into your lifestyle and habits to look for those root causes—those 100 things that can turn on this memory-shattering disease.

But you have to start NOW!

CHAPTER FIVE REFERENCES

Bredesen DE. Reversing Cognitive Decline (Certification notes).

Darion, J., Leigh, M. (1965). The Impossible Dream. On Man of La Mancha [CD] New York, N.Y.: Sam Fox Publishing Company.

Bredesen DE, Amos EC, Canick J, et al. Reversal of cognitive decline in Alzheimer's disease. Aging (Albany NY). 2016; 8(6):1250-1258. doi:10.18632/aging.100981.

Smits LL, van Harten AC, Pijnenburg YA, et al. Trajectories of cognitive decline in different types of dementia. Psychological Medicine. 2015 Apr; 45(5):1051-9.

Deng W, Aimone JB, Gage FH. New neurons and new memories: how does adult hippocampal neurogenesis affect learning and memory? Nature reviews Neuroscience. 2010; 11(5):339-350. doi:10.1038/nrn2822.

Johnson R, Halder G. The two faces of Hippo: targeting the Hippo pathway for regenerative medicine and cancer treatment. Nature Reviews Drug Discovery. 2014; 13(1):63-79. doi:10.1038/nrd4161.

Park M, Salgado JM, Ostroff L, et al. Plasticity-Induced Growth of Dendritic Spines by Exocytic Trafficking from Recycling Endosomes. Neuron. 2006; 52(5): 817-830. doi:10.1016/j.neuron.2006.09.040.

Weintraub S, Wicklund AH, Salmon DP. The Neuropsychological Profile of Alzheimer Disease. Cold Spring Harbor Perspectives in Medicine. 2012; 2(4):a006171. doi:10.1101/cshperspect.a006171.

CHAPTER SIX

RE-CHARGE SUPPORT

Today, we're exploring a new world—one that I guarantee you've never been to before! It is a new world of Extreme Support Teams. You see...

Operation Hope's goal is to create robust support teams committed to helping people with cognitive decline to live a fuller, more vibrant life.

To do this we *have* to be different, and our first step towards being different is to re-charge support.

What do I mean by "re-charge"? Well, when you connect your cell phone to a power source, it re-charges your cell phone, so it works again. The power source supports, strengthens, and electrifies the cellphone... The same thing happens with a support group when we re-charge it. By connecting the support group to a power source, we are strengthened.

Remember, support means: "to carry, protect, lift up, bear, endure, suffer with, strengthen, and fight for... together."

Support in Action, is a collective, a community, a village, a team, a group of like-minded people who together support a cause to carry, protect, lift up, strengthen, and fight for an individual's cause.

I had a patient named Claire, who had fast progressing Alzheimer's. Our goal was to slow down her cognitive decline, restore memory, and boost nutrition again so that her body could re-charge.

Claire shares with us a song that speaks of what we must do to recharge support:

O lift me up on Your wings.

Let me soar while my heart sings.

O lift me up on Your wings

so I can see what Your love brings.

Words and music: Jon Pourroy

Reference: Exodus 19:4

And while Claire cannot say this for herself right now, we can almost hear her say from within:

Yes, lift me up... see me, hear me, talk with me, touch me, take my hand... hold me. Oh, lift me up on your wings... My wings are tired, bruised, and broken. I'm so lonely.... Inside of me I scream, "Hello, are you there?" I am still here, but you walk away without hearing. You do not hear me because now I speak differently... silently... from deep inside of me...

I still burn with life! Do not push me away! I'm not done yet! I'm just caged in this cruel remember-less cocoon. Yet I remember. Oh, how I remember.

Please, do not push me away. Lift me up on your wings and let me soar. I want to see what your love brings... Push power into my wings.

[Ann L. Johnson, for Claire]

Claire, and all of those we love who are experiencing cognitive decline are asking us to learn the "language of the silent." But, what is this "language of the silent" and how do we learn it?

The Language of the Silent is a new language—one without alphabet or consonants; it is a whole life expressed in the twinkle of an eye or the splash of a teardrop.

This Language of the Silent is an amphitheater for the 8 Senses within you and it is a language that can be heard, felt, and seen. Yet, it goes deeper than where normal languages go—it has deeper roots that go all the way to your cells and your DNA.

THE LANGUAGE OF THE SILENT IS THE DNA OF HOPE.

The Language of the Silent is the language of being there for someone; it is the language of time well spent—because it takes your precious time to learn how to "talk" again with your loved one.

The Language of the Silent is the language of champions and heroes because this is what it takes to restore hope. And hope is a two-way street where there is hope for the patient but there is also hope for the collective.

When you see the Language of the Silent in action it is electrifying and it re-charges hope.

This is why we start Extreme Support Teams, to push power into those wings once again. So, as you start your own Extreme Support group, keep the following in your vision and your mind:

Your wings, my wings, our wings! A winged vision, living in freedom, uncaged, and soaring!

To start your own Extreme Support group, consider the following information:

WHAT IS A SUPPORT GROUP?

1. Like-minded people who have a common riveting cause.

2. People who want to work together in a place where everybody is equal, including the person with the cognitive decline.

3. A group of people who want to learn and share the good times and help carry the load in bad times, knowing that everyone will experience both the good and the bad in so many shades throughout their unbelievable wellness journeys.

WHO DO WE ASK TO JOIN OUR SUPPORT GROUP?

1. Family, friends, neighbors.

2. Practitioners like nutritionists, health coaches, massage therapists, nurses, and the client's physician (many of these licensed practitioners do come if asked, but you have to ask).

Did you know practitioners love to see support around individuals? In fact, it really catches our attention! If the phrase "build it and they'll come" has any relevance, it is here with practitioners. Show us and odds are, we will join you!

WHERE TO MEET WITH A SUPPORT GROUP?

1. Familiar places are always better. People love their culture, their special places, where they recognize home aromas—and this is deeper than we know—these aromas turn on comfort, relaxation, they open up minds and lower people's barriers so that a person's true self can emerge!

2. The family home. The family home works for some, while others prefer the privacy of a community or church location.

3. Recreation areas like parks or open spaces.

In regard to a meeting place, you are only limited by your creativity and safe access to the meeting area. Always consider safety, home or building access, ease of walkways outside the building and inside, restroom access, and handicap accessibility. (Remove any throw rugs because they can be fall hazards!)

As you are thinking about the logistics of a support group—**keep it simple.**

Some just start by asking one person… And just by starting you are stimulating the growth of new neurons! Anytime we learn, get curious, start a new project… we grow new neurons. **So, let's start!**

But are you willing to stand up and say with, or for, your mother, father, wife, husband, partner, friend, or yourself, "I believe we will get better. I believe. I just need to start"?

So as you stand up and start your support group, remember, there are **three rules to follow:**

THREE RULES FOR SUPPORT

1. We support each other, no matter what. We support each other ferociously, and we refuse to be refused.

2. We believe we can change the course of cognitive decline for the better, together. This is our power belief!

3. This power-belief drives positive changes within the group and individual.

We have been hopeless, with the wrong power-belief. We have been told there is nothing we can do to change this decline. But since 2014, we know better, and we have won the Cognitive Performance Olympics with many.

Yes, we can change cognitive decline to cognitive performance— if we work as a team.

If we change our belief from "No, we can't" to "Yes, we can," we can build hope, and hope re-charges support.

We must understand that a support team is essential because change and re-charging support happens on so many levels… community, group, family, individual, and all the way to our cells and our DNA.

So, take the time to re-think your beliefs about cognitive decline.

Together, we can change the face of cognitive decline and re-charge cognitive performance—supporting people who want to get their life and memory back! This is my promise!

So, reach out and start. Ask people to join your support group. I want to see what your love brings.

HOW TO ENGAGE OR POWER UP YOUR SUPPORT TEAMS

Next, let's discuss **how to engage or power up your support teams**, your belief team.

The root word "engage" means "to pledge, to involve, to enter into combat."

As we engage in this very unique support group, we are powered by the collective—being powered by a collective will take on a transformational meaning, but first, let's make sure we are all on the same page with our AIM.

Our AIM is to prevent, slow down, and even reverse cognitive decline.

We are the pioneers, here! We are facing a formidable enemy—a disease that recently had a 0% success rate. Together, we can change this number, but **we must engage support to fight this disease**. No one can do this alone... No one... So, **as a collective, we need to engage the 8 Circles of Support.**

We will NOT change the course of cognitive decline to cognitive incline without:

1. fighting for each other

2. fighting for ourselves

3. fighting for our inside cellular wellness.

Believe me, it is a battle. I have been doing this for 40 years with clients on all spectrums of illness; from strokes to accidents in shock trauma, to strength training with wheelchair/walker-bound clients, to decreasing Parkinson's symptoms with lifestyle, to healthy aging and helping 80-year-olds walk, run, and travel again. And does it ever motivate me to continue to fight for clients who progress so far… as to leave the walker behind and cruise the world.

I've seen this happen again and again, and now I want this for you, for all of you with various levels of cognitive decline. Let's learn to fight for each other and support each other. Yes, it is an uphill battle, **but together we can!**

REAL LIFE EXAMPLE

I had a client who was working with me to stop being hungry all the time, lose weight, boost memory, and learn how to smile again.

His overall AIM was to "stop my hands from shaking." So, we did his M.A.P. and we tested his cellular metabolism and genomics. Then, we switched his nutrition plan, added more absorbable protein and amino acids, slowly added olive oil and fish oils along with acetyl-L-carnitine (fat carrier into the brain and cells), and a few other things.

With the help of his support team (he shared his AIM with them), collectively they ate better, worked out and walked more together, and measured progress together… After six months, this is what happened: during his 6-month visit to his neurologist, the doctor opens up the door and stares at him. Looking at his client's chart, he says, "Are you Mister…?"

He did not recognize him! My client had lost weight, was smiling, laughing with face and feet no longer swollen, and even better, steadier hands!

I love these true stories. Especially when they are my clients who are doing their work and engaging their support team to help them. This is when we know hope is working and creating its nutrients of belief and support.

NOTE: Share your AIM or goal with others. This gives more power to everyone and then your support team becomes part of your jury—convicting you to a higher level of success and health and wellness.

Now, let's go deeper and talk about the 8 Circles of Support, which are truly amazing success builders.

In the 8 Circles of Support, **the goal is for all the circles to be concentric and fit within each other**. In real life, this rarely happens; but with this concept, we now have a measurable way to check on the progress of a support team.

Look at the 8 Circles of Support Anatomy. Each of them represents:

- Circle 1: Your microbiome.

- Circle 2: Your cells and your metabolism.

- Circle 3: Your mind and your beliefs.

- Circle 4: Your inner support circle (most trusted and valued family and friends—people who "refuse to be refused," who will fight ferociously for you and move mountains, so you can get better).

- Circle 5: Your helping support team (the people who want to help by doing "things" such as shopping, meals, transportation. Consider them the administrative assistant of the Support Team).

- Circle 6: Family and friends who visit and touch base often but are not involved in full with the support team.

- Circle 7: Practitioners, mentors, and partners in care.

- Circle 8: Your community: where you shop, dine, work out, etc.

These 8 circles are your jury—the men and women who will convict you to a higher level of wellness.

HOW TO GROW SUPPORT IN A GROUP?

To grow support in a group, sometimes you just need to start and then get the message out. Yes, just start. Change what you do, "get out of line," do something different, try something new.

If, in the beginning, your team has only one person, fret not! Pick up your shield and fight on! More will join, but what is missing is your voice. Yes, your voice.

And your voice is your belief. Your voice is hope in action.

CHAPTER SIX REFERENCE

Johnson AL. The DNA of Hope. Christiana, PA. Ann-Louise Johnson, 2018.

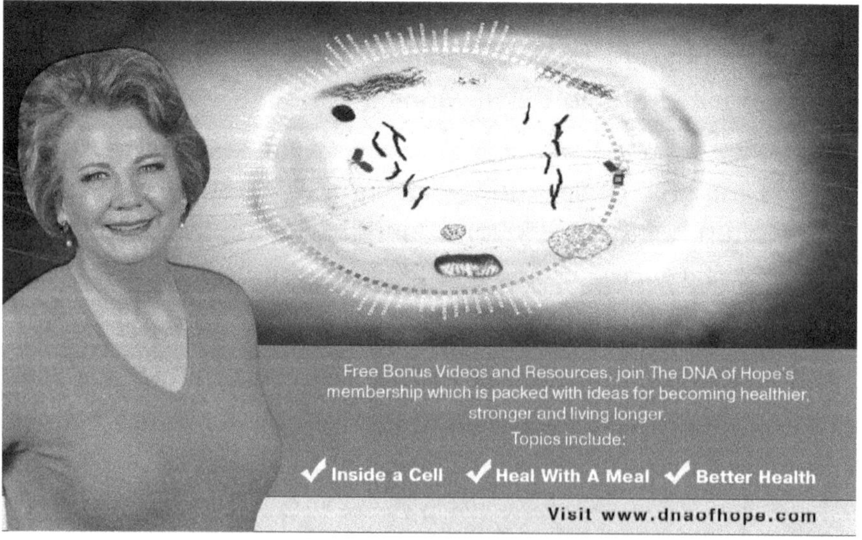

CHAPTER SEVEN

MOVE ME MOTIVATION

Struggle has so many benefits. Being in a struggle causes you to work harder and say, "I can" or "I can't."

Struggle can motivate us to work harder, be more, do more.

Yet, we still need support from others and the strength that comes from within.

I like to share a story about a rose that illustrates the benefits of the struggle.

The rose struggled alone. No one cared. The rose's caregiver had left her, not giving instructions to water, feed, and prize this beauty—there would be no one to smell it, to touch it, to talk to it, to listen to it, and to watch the bees taste and spread the rose's sweetness. Oh, no one cared for this rose. No one remembered it. No one supported it.

But, wait! Look at the tiny rosebud right by the larger rose. Something thrives in the midst of the struggle...

And that is how my mother regenerated her rosebushes into grand-prize show quality roses. Those California boys would come to Arizona where she lived, and they would say, "Hmm, we can beat her." But my mother knew the secret of the rose.

Struggles have so many benefits—struggle blossoms strength.

And this is how my mother won the king of show again and again. I remember walking with her in her garden, hand-in-hand, as she shared with me, *"Listen to the rose. Talk to it. Give it more life by touching it, smelling it, and enjoying its fragrance, and learn the secret of the rose. Roses grow to be stunning when pruned hard. Stress them a little, talk to them, and listen to their secrets like I did, then stand back and be amazed."*

I was already amazed at my mother, but I became even more amazed when I discovered that she had the genes for super rose-smelling. Yes, there are genes for that. As dear Rose said so eloquently, "Move me. Astonish me. Unnerve me. Delight my eyes and my brain afterward, if you care to."

Roses moved and astonished my mother. She delighted in them.

Her eyes and her smile just lit up. Her brain lit up whenever a rose's fragrance wafted. She nursed them to become stronger and healthier with love, olive oil, and nutrients.

So now, **how can we take the principle of the rose and apply it to our family and friends with cognitive decline?** Oh, they are our Roses, often living through their decline alone and afraid. Rose is unable to say what she needs. Our family and friends with this disease have become more afraid, and fear turns off an individual's ability to learn.

Rose gets worse as people stay away. They can't talk to her, they say. Rose's world gets smaller and smaller, darker and more isolated. Her 8 Senses get dull from lack of use, and, yes, when the 8 Senses dull, brain growth slows and slows and stops. Neurons stop growing. Synapses stop firing. And neurons and synapses separate from each other. They curl up into a ball. The signals are now muffled. It's too long a distance to hear that signal. So, they become silent. Signals are not heard inside. There is no wiring and no firing. Just quiet.

Oh, is someone listening? Is someone out there learning the Language of the Silent? Wait! There is hope, still, hope, unwilling to accept the life dished this way. Someone in the family circle of friends stands up and says, "Is there something I can do for Rose to help her be more alive again, to help her be with us again?"

But we have found that **struggle motivates**. And when, in the midst of struggle, despair, and frustration, someone stands up with the courage to still hope and say "we can," the hearts of many become motivated again.

Even a single person becoming motivated—and I've seen this over and over again—can turn the tide.

You see, **motivation can be so infectiously healthy.** So, show up. Be there. Learn. Give. And stand up for the Roses of this world!

Now, let's analyze what happens in the brain when it faces a struggle, as illustrated with the rose. As we journey into the brain, we will begin to discover a whole new world—and oh, what a wonderful journey it will be! We're also going to look at the brain structure of fragrance and relate it to our world of sensing, hearing, motivation, fear, pain, plasticity, learning, and regrowth.

As you have that fragrance that you love, whether it's a person, a spice, or a flower, let's start relating it back to those 8 Senses that we learned earlier.

Smell. Smell works in multiple brain areas. It works in the olfactory bulb, the prefrontal cortex, the thalamus, and the hippocampal area right behind the eyes.

Memory. Memory works in the prefrontal cortex and the hippocampal area. There are many other areas, but we're trying to keep it simple here.

Vision. Vision works in the occipital area, at the back of the brain.

Motivation. Motivation works in the anterior cingulate area—we'll focus here a little bit later.

Emotions and **fear.** Fear that we have someone standing up to help someone when no one else will. That fear evolves right around the amygdala.

Plasticity and flexibility occur when we learn and stress our brains. Therefore, in your support groups, it's important to use the 8 Senses through things like tasting, feeling, smelling, hearing, remembering, etc. Think of a synapse as a space. Learning and working our brains causes electrical signals to start building back and forth between the neurons and synapses. This brain exercise also works in our mitochondria, those energy powerhouses that work within your cells and promote life within you.

Curiosity and motivation are tied together right in your mitochondria. There are 5,000 of these little organelles in every single heart cell. I call them mito-hope because they are the center of our hope. Curiosity is what will get you or your loved one out of that cognitive decline.

Moisture. Every single cell needs fluid. The cell membranes need to be fluid. They need to be a liquid type thing, and the olfactory neurons and connections all need fluid and moisture to function.

Support. Neurons, dendrites, and synapses—all of the things that connect us—need to be connected with support.

"WHAT DOES MY BRAIN DO?"

Well, it connects your ears, for one. It balances your head on your shoulders, and, yes, there's a sense that it does a lot more things. Unfortunately, some people's brains have grown smaller and smaller and smaller through life. **However, as we learn more, our brain can grow**. If we live in fear, our brain shrinks. **If we live in love, our brain grows. If we enjoy learning and curiosity, our brain grows.**

Next, we're going to concentrate on growing the anterior cingulate area. **The anterior cingulate area is the center of motivation**. Sometimes, we call it "rewards," "surprise," "conflict," so on and so forth. However, I find that those terms are all kind of boring.

The anterior cingulate is underneath the brain. It's a whole area that people are wondering about; what it actually does—but the reality is that it does so much!

As we electrically stimulate the anterior cingulate in clients, it promotes in them a will to persevere. What does this mean? It means that **they begin to have the desire to overcome a challenge.**

Let's get back to motivation. At its very core, then, **what is motivation?**

Motivation is the internal force that prompts a person to take action. It is what gives you the power when you are at your weakest. It's a determination, a drive, or pursuit of a goal or aim, no matter what.

Remember that. Refuse to be refused in the face of obstacles, boredom, fatigue, stress, and illness!

Motivation is our inner power and our inner sweat. It's what infuses hope all the way to our DNA. Did you know motivation has a three-dimensional form to it, as in structure, function, and behavior? We learned what structure, function, and behavior are in a previous lesson. Structure answers the question, **"Do I have a chance?"** I further define chance as a challenge for my clients, a symptom.

I quantify this challenge by asking my clients two questions:

1. What is your most important aim or goal that you want to accomplish in life—what's your big sky goal?

2. What are three symptoms you want to get rid of?

QUESTION ONE: THE AIM.

The answer to question one lets me know *how motivated they are*. An individual's aim is important. Some people say, "I want to change the world by..." (you can finish the sentence). Some people say, "I just want to learn how to do this." Another one will say, "I just want to feel again." **You can actually tell where a person is in their life and health by their aim**.

The aim also hints at their strengths or their weaknesses and their support system. If I have a person who's tired and worn out, and their support system is nonexistent, then I know their anterior cingulate is also worn out. So, **by bringing in supportive people I can help build their system back into**

existence. Again, I'm awakening that anterior cingulate and bringing back hope.

QUESTION TWO: THE SYMPTOMS.

The answer to question two allows me to better define our job together as a partnership, to read the symptoms so that the client can reach his or her aim. I've had clients want to get rid of brain fog or sadness so deep it can be felt in your fingernails. Others mention constipation, or a burning pain in their feet and hands, or slow thinking, or a lack of appetite.

Motivation equals move me, delight me, get rid of my symptoms, let me feel again, remember again. **Remember, we have to believe in the power of our own dreams before we will stand for someone else's dreams**. We have to build our own motivation to reach our dream.

The following information I am about to share is new information that took a significant amount of time and research to find. I don't think anybody in the world has heard this, and you will be amongst the first to read about it.

To grow that anterior cingulate area, you need to dance. You need to delight your brain.

Move your curiosity. It doesn't matter if you dance on the dance floor, if you dance in your wheelchair, or if you dance in bed. **Just move that body**. We are made to move. Delight your brain. Move and listen. Sit still and concentrate. Do some brain games. Move me. Astonish me. Unnerve me. Delight my eyes and brain afterward, if you care to. Be there. Learn the secret of the rose!

Before we continue, let us remember the **Three Rules for Support**.

1. We support each other no matter what. We support each other ferociously and we refuse to be refused.

2. We believe we can change the course of cognitive decline for the better together. This is our power belief.

3. This power belief drives positive change within the group and the individual as previously discussed; it also drives change in every blueprint layer of your timeline and your M.A.P.—your Health Blueprint, your Cellular Blueprint, and your DNA and Genes Blueprint.

THE POWER OF BELIEF

Let us continue talking about belief. We first discussed belief in the 8 Pillar lesson. We know that **belief changes us at each layer of our M.A.P.** Note that a power belief, a positive belief, can recharge our mitochondria, and our mitochondria are the center of hope. We call this our "mito-hope."

The power of any support team is the power of their belief.

That's so important I want you to read it again: the power of any support team is the power of their belief. I want your support team to believe that we can change the course of cognitive decline, because we can.

Watch your beliefs, they are powerful.

WHAT HAPPENS WHEN YOU BELIEVE

This is what happens when you believe: **miracles happen.** When we believe we can change things; when we have support;

when we turn on that motivation again, **change happens and life blossoms.**

Be there. Be the support person for the people that you love. Feel their pain.

I remember one of my clients. He had cognitive decline and was often unable to find words or do math. He was a salesman, but now he could hardly even think! He had three symptoms he wanted to go away; he had pain in his hands (they were shaking, Parkinson's-like), he was on an emotional roller coaster (he would be up one minute, and way down the next, sometimes even crying), and he had severe constipation. His gut microbiome—which is the sum total of the bacteria within you—was mostly bad bacteria. And this actually turned on illness. (Your gut microbiome is about nine-tenths of you. We need to pay attention to it.)

So, my client had significant problems with fat malabsorption, and he also had genetic challenges with cellular repair and poor glutathione levels. That is your intracellular antioxidant that repairs the cell. It is the major one, and he could not make it. Food and sleep were the two major pillars that he was having problems with. His aim was that he just wanted to feel again.

He was that low. **But within six months of working with me, his hands were steady, his gut was functioning, he increased his protein levels, and his body turned on repair.** He is back at the computer doing his sales again, and he's functioning. His aim has changed, he is making money again, he's got his support, and he loves his wife again. **These are the things that matter.**

Another client had an APOE4 +/- gene. APOE4 +/- gene is one of the major genes that can lead a person down the trajectory to

Alzheimer's. There are statistical probabilities if you're a plus-minus, or a plus-plus. I will not get too into this, but if you have the APOE4 as either +/+ or +/-, you have got to pay attention: the statistics don't matter!

This person was a writer and had been experiencing cognitive decline for five years, so the writing suffered. The three symptoms he wanted to go away were: extreme fatigue (he was spending most of his time in bed), headaches, and he was forgetting things too much.

Cellularly, he had poor gut absorption and particularly, poor protein absorption. He needed hydrochloric acid (you need hydrochloric acid in order to absorb protein). He had a red flair on his cheeks and his nose, and if you looked closely, he had broken blood vessels called rosacea (rosacea is often a sign of low hydrochloric acid). He had lots of nausea and a tremendous amount of gas, particularly an hour after every meal. His mitochondria were wimpy. They needed all of the B vitamins; B1, B2, B3, B5, B7, B9, B12. He had very poor fat absorption.

He ate a lot of sugar. His glucose levels were much too high, and his hemoglobin A1C, which should be 5 or less was at 11.5. This means that his red blood cells were toasted in sugar. Regarding his pillars, he had zero motivation, zero support, and his food was excess sugar and very high carbohydrates, so he also had lots of allergies. His aim in life—he still had one, believe it or not—was that he wanted to write a book that would change the world. Would you get behind somebody like that? I **was ready.**

Nine months later, **he is writing again, and he is on a mitochondrial core diet**. That's a particular one we'll be using for many of you. Not eating after 6:00 PM until breakfast again at 9:00 AM is important. You know what that does? Your mitochondria, those little fellas in the cell, they divide. You want two of them, and to get there, don't eat so much. My client is also exercising again, walking three miles a day. Not much, but much better than nothing. He's challenging his brain with his new book. He is motivated again.

What changed? He got support from his family and his neighbors. What happened? Now, he is passing it on. He is providing support for others.

Together we can change the face of cognitive decline and recharge cognitive performance, supporting people who want to get their life and memory back. We can. We can. We can—together.

CHAPTER SEVEN REFERENCES

Pelowski M, Markey PS, Forster M, Gerger G, Leder H. Move me, astonish me… delight my eyes and brain: The Vienna Integrated Model of top-down and bottom-up processes in Art Perception (VIMAP) and corresponding affective, evaluative, and neurophysiological correlates. Physics of Life Reviews. 2017 Jul; 21:80-125. doi: 10.1016/j.plrev.2017.02.003. Epub 2017 Feb 27.

Sherwin E, Rea K, Dinan TG, Cryan JF. A gut (microbiome) feeling about the brain. Current Opinion in Gastroenterology. 2016 Mar; 32(2). doi: 10.1097/MOG.0000000000000244.

Ebitz RB, Hayden BY. Dorsal anterior cingulate: a Rorschach test for cognitive neuroscience. Nature Neuroscience. 2016 Oct; 19(10): 1278-1279.

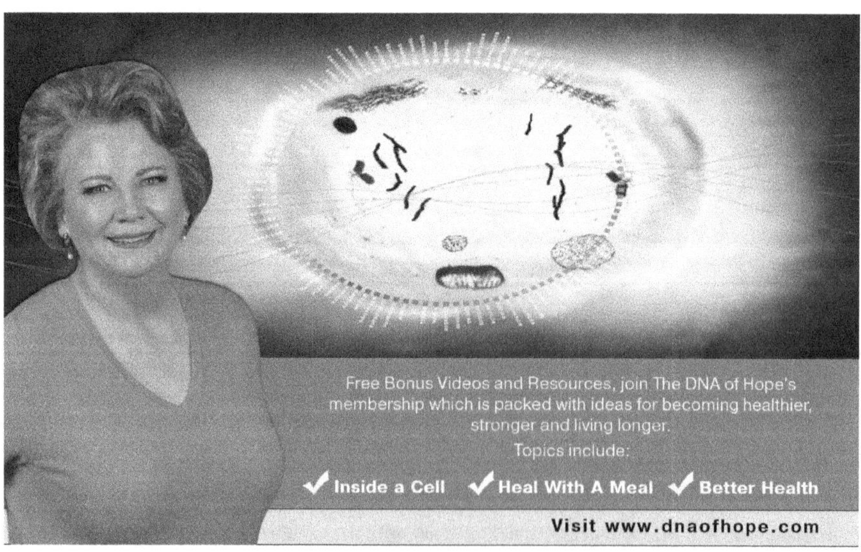

CHAPTER EIGHT

THE ENERGY OF FOOD

1. THE LION STORY—DOES YOUR FOOD MAKE YOU ROAR?

I was recently at a zoo during the lions' feeding time. I was mesmerized, watching these majestic creatures—pacing steadily with bold, proud steps. But the best part of the experience was watching—and hearing—their response to the food they were about to receive. With senses awakened and on alert, all the lions would simultaneously begin to let out deep, loud roars… It was magnificent!

I'm not exactly sure why lions roar while feeding—maybe it's social communication? Maybe it's their way to protect their meal? Or perhaps even appetite stimulation?

Whatever the reason, the experience got me thinking…

Does *my* food make *me* roar?

And in asking myself this, my mind immediately responded—yes… **but *only* if I am eating certain types of foods**. There are so many reasons why we eat as humans in this first-world society, beyond the biological necessity… ***We eat to socialize, to celebrate, to honor traditions, to create pleasure, to try new experiences, to soothe pain, to pacify loneliness, and to overall connect with ourselves and others.***

With so many opportunities to eat, so many types of modern food available to us, and so many packaged, processed, and scientifically-engineered food products on the market—combined with a fast and/or even ultra-fast pace of life—it's easy to fall into patterns, to not actively think about the food choices we are making, and to end up inadvertently poisoning our precious cells.

And, since eating is such a common, every-day part of our existence, **we tend to forget how powerful it really is**. We take it for granted… and become a bit mindless sometimes in our relationship with it. Even when we know certain foods are loaded with sugar, preservatives, or the big one—high fructose corn syrup—we lose perspective that we are actually putting these toxins inside our body, and into our cells. But the truth is:

Every single substance we put into our body is absorbed and becomes a part of who we are.

The old adage—"you are what you eat"—is not just a saying. This is legitimately exactly what is happening, deep inside your body, with every bite.

As I was leaving the zoo, I saw a mother with two children in tow. She was feeding her smallest child, who was not yet even walking, a soda. This is so commonplace in our society that many people don't think anything of it. And I am sure this well-intentioned mother **does not *really* understand how damaging soda can be**, especially to developing cells. However, **once you know how poisonous high-fructose corn syrup is to our bodies, it's hard to look at it the same**. The can of soda begins to look like what it is—a can of poison. And then seeing it fed to a small child… becomes painful to watch.

It's often hard to recognize the true power of food until you eliminate something toxic from your diet, and then first-hand experience the difference.

Because until then… many people simply don't know what they don't know. They may be experiencing health challenges, fatigue, and/or a lack of focus. However, they attribute these short-comings to "just what happens as you get older," or a genetic predisposition, or something "they just have to deal with." Even worse, and likely even more common, **they don't even realize there is a problem at all.**

Many people have deviated so far away from their body's natural state of optimum health, that they don't even remember what feeling vibrant, energized, and full of life feels like anymore. They have forgotten that they even have a roar… buried somewhere inside.

When I am eating colorful fruits and vegetables and full, flavorful, vegetable soups cooked with meat… I can feel my cells come to life. It's like every cell inside of me is shouting, "Yes! Thank you!" This is what makes me "roar."

Eating optimum, nutrient-rich, and cell-nourishing food stimulates super energy, a clear brain, a strong memory, and ultimately… sustained happiness.

So today… I challenge you to really think about your current state of being, in connection with each bite of food you have recently put in your body, and honestly ask yourself:

"Does my food make me roar?"

2. FOOD IS MEDICINE

Food, at its core level, **is actually a computer-like coded package of information that is unwrapped, digested, and then used by your cells to either heal or slay you**, as Dr. Mark Hyman would say. In the form of carbohydrates, fats, and proteins, these "nutrient-codes" are delivered and processed throughout your body. In turn, your cells will readily use the nutrient-dense components of each package as building blocks for your body's growth and healing. Or, they will be forced to attack, enclose, or work to eliminate anything that they don't recognize or cannot use.

Unfortunately, our H.A.D., or Horrible American Diet, also coined by Dr. Mark Hyman, is packed with much of the latter.

The average American meal is largely comprised of cow's milk, white bread, flour-based pastries, processed cheese, and processed meat—all of which are taxing to the body.

And even though we live in an era in which cases of chronic illnesses and auto-immune diseases are continuously on the rise, we continue to create and consume new "designer-foods" that our cells and genes are unable to process—and in doing so, we sadly continue to exacerbate the problem.

We have to stop the madness. We have to take a step back and realize—with paramount importance—that our food choices really, really matter.

Several years ago, I witnessed a social worker's success with incarcerated criminals. **She was able to turn around several prisoners' aggressive behavior simply by changing their food**. The same results have been replicated and studied by a variety of researchers. A prison trial at the Aylesbury jail in London showed that when prisoners were fed multivitamins, minerals, and essential fatty acids, the number of violent offenses they committed fell by 37%. The clinician in charge of this study, a man named Joseph Hibbeln, was not surprised by the results—in fact, he said it was predictable if you understand the biochemistry of the brain and the biophysics of the brain cell membrane.

Our brains and our bodies *need* quality nutrients to operate and function at their best.

The power of food is real—it is our body's best friend and best medicine. As Hippocrates, the great Greek physician known as the Father of Modern Medicine, expressed back in about 400 BC, "Let food be thy medicine, and medicine be thy food."

3. FOOD PROVIDES BUILDING BLOCKS FOR OUR BODY

Think of each bite of natural food you eat as a building block, and every bite of processed, packaged, or scientifically engineered food as a wrecking ball. Because your body doesn't recognize these modern foods, it has to use your precious energy to eliminate or store them—usually by burying them in your fat cells or within cell walls.

When you think about what you eat, I want you to begin **visualizing the effect your food is having inside your body.**

4. WE NEED TO BE PROACTIVE—MARKETERS WON'T DO IT FOR US

As difficult and/or overwhelming as it may seem at first to guard your body against all of the processed junk that is now out there and to fill it with real nutrients and amino acids that it can use—**this task is up to you. Your life and long-term well-being depend on it.** In fact, if you are already suffering from cognitive decline, this really is not an option—it's a must.

Everywhere you turn in our modern world, we are being solicited to buy engineered, processed, sugary, and unhealthy foods—and some of them even taste really good. Marketers will print anything on a package if they think it might persuade us to eat it.

But just because it says that it's "organic" or "healthy" or "low-carb" or "gluten-free" on the package does not mean that it's good for you.

You have to take the time to read the label, to look at the actual ingredients, to evaluate the levels of sodium, sugar, and trans-fats inside before gracing any food with the gift of traveling inside your body. This requires a keen diligence, a steadfast standard, and an unwavering commitment to providing your body with quality foods.

5. HEAL WITH A MEAL©

So yes—in our world today, the odds are stacked against you when it comes to regularly eating and preparing healthy food. However, **once you know what the foods you consume are actually doing inside your body, you will never be able to look at them the same way again.**

And to make a change toward more healing foods, I encourage you to simply start small.

I call this philosophy, **"Heal with a Meal"**©. Changing all of your food habits drastically at one time can be overwhelming—maybe even to the point where it sets you back, even from a biological perspective. Every time you change the foods you eat, the bacteria in your gut change as well, which could have negative consequences if you do it too quickly. So, rather than throwing everything in your kitchen out today, **focus instead on setting yourself up for success slowly by working to create just one meal every day comprised of only healthy protein, fats, and carbs.**

Then, in a couple of sessions—we will provide you with the tools you need for a complete overhaul—including shopping lists, recipes, and practical tips to surround yourself with only life-giving, energy-creating foods.

I leave you with this—if you remember nothing else from this session, please remember with each bite you take that food is medicine. Make it your medicine.

CHAPTER EIGHT REFERENCES

Zeng Y, Li Y, Yang J, et al. Therapeutic Role of Functional Components in Alliums for Preventive Chronic Disease in Human Being. Evidence-Based Complementary and Alternative Medicine. 2017; 2017: 9402849.

Stangl D, Thuret S. Impact of diet on adult hippocampal neurogenesis. Genes & Nutrition. 2009; 4(4):271-282. doi: 10.1007/s12263-009-0134-5.

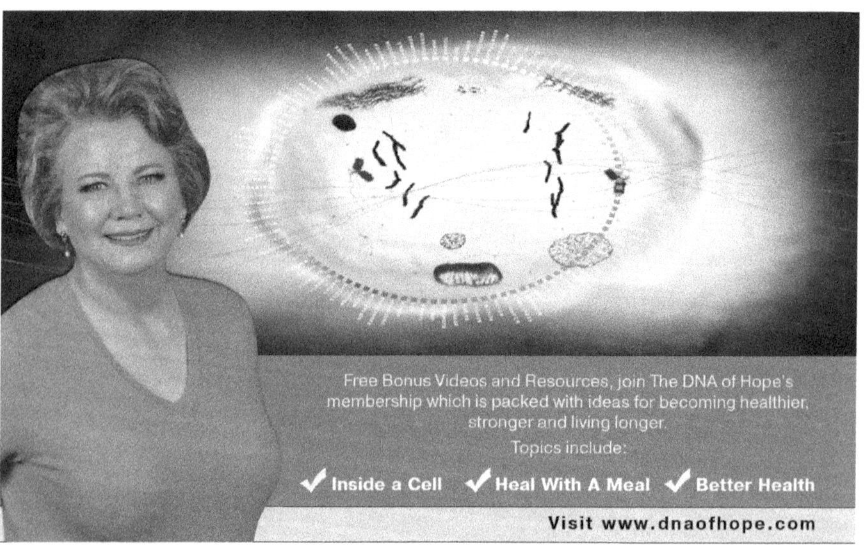

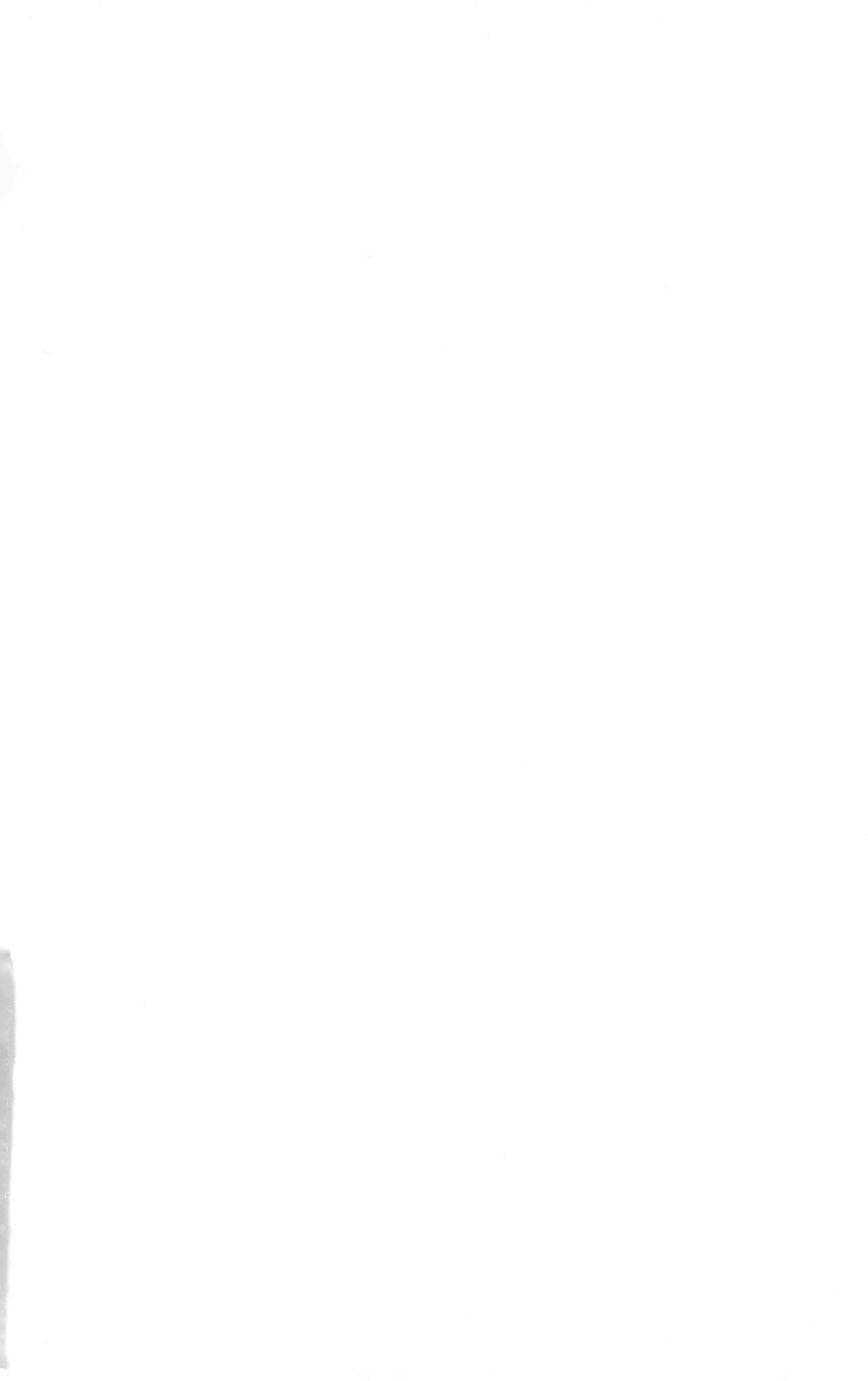